Spanish Phrasebook for Medical and Social Services Professionals

Jarvis Lebredo Lebredo

Houghton Mifflin Company
Boston New York

Director, Modern Language Programs:
E. Kristina Baer
Development Manager: Beth Kramer
Associate Development Editor:
Rafael Burgos-Mirabal
Editorial Assistant: Nasya Laymon
Manufacturing Manager: Florence Cadran
Associate Marketing Manager:
Tina Crowley-Desprez

Printed in the U.S.A.

ISBN: 0-395-96308-7

456789-EW-06 05 04 03 02

Preface

Four pocket phrasebooks now accompany the successful *Basic Spanish Grammar (BSG)* communication and career manual series. Each provides handy reference word lists to assist students of Spanish for specific career purposes and professionals who use Spanish in the workplace, reinforcing the practical approach that this program has offered to Spanish learners for the past twenty years.

The *BSG* series includes a core grammar textbook, two communication manuals (the introductory *Getting Along in Spanish* and the higher-level *Spanish for Communication*) and five career manuals: *Spanish for Business and Finance, Spanish for Medical Personnel, Spanish for Law Enforcement, Spanish for Social Services,* and *Spanish for Teachers.* When used in combination with the *BSG* grammar textbook, the career manuals teach students the basic structures of Spanish and the vocabulary pertaining to specific professions.

As their titles indicate, the phrasebooks include the terms and phrases that appear in six manuals:

Phrasebook for Getting Along in Spanish
Spanish Phrasebook for Business, Finance, and Everyday Communication

Spanish Phrasebook for Medical and Social Services Professionals
Spanish Phrasebook for Law Enforcement and Social Services Professionals

Since many learners of Spanish for specific careers are English speakers, the phrasebooks include Spanish–English and English–Spanish listings. Designed for use in the office or in the field, these phrasebooks will provide a convenient resource for professionals who need a brief, portable guide to common Spanish words and phrases.

Abbreviations Used in This Book

The following abbreviations are used in this phrasebook.

adj.	adjective
adv.	adverb
coll.	colloquial
f.	feminine noun
fam.	familiar
form.	formal
inf.	infinitive
m.	masculine noun
Méx.	Mexico
pl.	plural
pron.	pronoun
sing.	singular

Spanish–English

A

a to, at
  — **casa** home
  — **la derecha** to the right
  — **la izquierda** to the left
  — **la semana** weekly, per week
  — **largo plazo** long term
  — **(la) medianoche** at midnight
  — **lo mejor** perhaps, maybe
  — **menudo** often
  — **nadie le importa.** It's nobody's business.
  — **partir de** starting with, as of
  — **plazos** in installments
  — **su alcance** within reach
  — **veces** sometimes
  — **ver.** Let's see.
abdomen (*m.*) abdomen
abierto(a) open
abogado(a) (*m., f.*) lawyer
aborto (*m.*) abortion
abrigo (*m.*) coat
abrir to open
absceso (*m.*) abscess
abstinencia (*f.*) abstinence
abuelo(a) (*m., f.*) grandfather; grandmother
abultamiento (*m.*) lump
abuso sexual (*m.*) sexual abuse
acabar de (+ *inf.*) to have just (done something), to have just (+ *past participle*)
acatarrado(a): estar — to have a cold
accesorio (*m.*) accessory

accidente (*m.*) accident
acción (*f.*) stock, share
aceite (*m.*) oil
aceptar to accept
acerca de about
acercarse to get close, to approach
acidez (*f.*) acidity, heartburn
ácido (*m.*) acid, LSD
acné (*m.*) acne
aconsejar to advise
acostar (o:ue) to put to bed
acostar(se) (o:ue) to lie down, to go to bed
actual present
actualmente currently, at the present time
acuerdo (*m.*) agreement
acusar to accuse
adelanto (*m.*) advance
adelgazar to lose weight
además besides, in addition
  — de besides, in addition to
adicional additional
adicto(a) addicted
adiós good-bye
adjetivo (*m.*) adjective
administrador(a) (*m., f.*) administrator
admisión (*f.*) admission
adolescente (*m., f.*) teenager
¿adónde? where (to)?
adulto(a) (*m., f.*) adult
afear to disfigure
afectar to affect
afeitar(se) to shave
afirmativo(a) affirmative
afuera outside

agarrar to take
agencia (*f.*) agency
agente de policía (*m., f.*) police officer
agradecer to thank
agua (*f.* but **el agua**) water
— **oxigenada** (*f.*) hydrogen peroxide
aguantar to hold, to stand, to tolerate, to bear
agudo(a) sharp, stabbing (*pain*)
aguja (*f.*) needle
agujero (*m.*) hole
ah oh
ahora now, at present
— **mismo** right now
— **no** not now, not at the present time
ahorita at present, now, right away (*Méx.*)
ahorros (*m. pl.*) savings
ahumado(a) smoked
aire (*m.*) air
— **acondicionado** (*m.*) air conditioning
ajá aha
al (a + el) to the; at the
— **año** yearly
— **contado** in cash, not on installments
— **cumplir... años** on becoming/turning . . . (years old)
— **día** a (per) day, daily
— **día siguiente** the next (following) day
— **dorso** over; on the back
— **final** at the end
— **mediodía** at midday (noon)
— **mes** monthly
— **pie de la página** at the bottom of the page
— **principio de** at the beginning
— **rato** a while later

alberca (*f.*) swimming pool (*Méx.*)
alcanzar to be enough
alcohol (*m.*) alcohol
alcohólico(a) alcoholic
Alcohólicos Anónimos Alcoholics Anonymous
alegrarse (de) to be glad
alergia (*f.*) allergy
alérgico(a) allergic
alfiler (*m.*) pin
alfombra (*f.*) rug
algo anything, something
  ¿— más? Anything else?
alguien somebody, someone, anybody, anyone
algún, alguno(a) any, some
  alguna vez ever
algunos(as) some
  algunas veces sometimes
aliento (*m.*) breath
alimentación (*f.*) food
alimentar to feed
alimento (*m.*) food, nourishment
aliviarse to feel better, to diminish (*a pain*)
allí there
almacenaje (*m.*) storage
almohada (*f.*) pillow
almorrana (*f.*) hemorrhoid
almorzar (o:ue) to have lunch
almuerzo (*m.*) lunch
alojamiento y las comidas (*m.*) room and board
alquiler (*m.*) rent
alrededor de around
alto(a) high, tall
alucinación (*f.*) hallucination

alumbramiento (*m.*) delivery
ama de casa (*f.* but **el ama**) housewife
amable kind
amamantar to feed, to nurse
amarillento(a) yellowish
amarillo(a) yellow
amarrar to tie
ambiente (*m.*) atmosphere
  la temperatura del — (*f.*) room temperature
ambulancia (*f.*) ambulance
ameno(a) pleasant, agreeable
americano(a) American
amígdalas (*f. pl.*) tonsils
amigdalitis (*f.*) tonsilitis
amigo(a) (*m., f.*) friend
ampolla (*f.*) blister
amputar to amputate
analgésicos (*m. pl.*) analgesics
análisis (*m.*) test, analysis
  — de sangre (*m.*) blood test
anciano(a) (*m., f.*) elderly man, elderly woman
andador (*m.*) walker
andar to go around, to walk
  — a gatas to crawl
anemia (*f.*) anemia
anémico(a) anemic
anestesia (*f.*) anesthesia
anestesiología (*f.*) anesthesiology
anestesiólogo(a) (*m., f.*) anethesiologist
aneurisma (*m.*) aneurysm
anfetamina (*f.*) amphetamine
angina (*f.*) angina
angioplastia, angioplastía (*f.*) angioplasty
angustia (*f.*) anxiety

anillo (*m.*) ring
ano (*m.*) anus
anoche last night
anotar to write down
ansiedad (*f.*) anxiety
anteanoche the night before last
anteayer the day before yesterday
anteojos (*m. pl.*) glasses, eyeglasses
anterior front, previous
antes (*adv.*) before, first
— **de** (*prep.*) before
antes de dormir before sleeping
antiácido (*m.*) antacid (medicine)
antibacteriano(a) antibacterial
antibiótico (*m.*) antibiotic
anticoagulante (*m.*) anticoagulant
anticonceptivo(a) (*adj.*) for birth control, contraceptive
antidepresivo (*m.*) antidepressant
antidiarreico (*m.*) antidiarrheic
antidroga antidrug
antiespasmódico (*m.*) antispasmodic
antihistamínico (*m.*) antihistamine
anual yearly
anualidad (*f.*) annuity
añadir to add
año (*m.*) year
aparato (*m.*) apparatus, instrument, system
— **intrauterino** (*m.*) I.U.D.
aparato eléctrico (*m.*) electrical (household) appliance
aparecer to appear
apartado postal (*m.*) post office box
apartamento (*m.*) apartment

apellido (*m.*) last name, surname
  — de soltera (*m.*) maiden name
apenas barely
apendicitis (*f.*) appendicitis
apestar to have a bad odor
apetito (*m.*) appetite
aplicar to apply
aprender to learn
apretar (e:ie) to press down, to be tight
aprobación (*f.*) approval
aprovechar to take advantage of
aquéllos(as) (*m., f.*) those
aquí here
  — está. Here it is.
  — mismo right here
  — tiene here is
árbol (*m.*) tree
archivo clínico (*m.*) medical records
arder to burn
ardor (*m.*) burning
arreglar to fix
arreglo (*m.*) arrangement
arrepentirse (e:ie) to regret, to feel sorry
arrestar to arrest
arriesgarse to risk
arrojar to throw up
arroz (*m.*) rice
arteria (*f.*) artery
articulación (*f.*) joint
artículo (*m.*) article
artificial artificial
artritis (*f.*) arthritis
ascensor (*m.*) elevator

aseguranza (*f.*) insurance (*Méx.*)
  — de salud (*f.*) health insurance (*Méx.*)
asegurarse to make sure
asentaderas (*f. pl.*) buttocks
asfixiar to suffocate
así like this, like that, that way, so
  — que so
  No es —. It is not that way.
asiento (*m.*) seat
asilo de ancianos (*m.*) home for the elderly
asimismo also
asistencia social (*f.*) social services
asistente (*m., f.*) assistant, helper
asistir a to attend
asma (*f.* but **el asma**) asthma
asmático(a) asthmatic
aspirina (*f.*) aspirin
astigmatismo (*m.*) astigmatism
asustarse to be scared, to be frightened
ataque (*m.*) seizure, attack
  — al corazón (*m.*) heart attack
atender (e:ie) to attend, to tend to, to take care of, to wait on
atragantarse to choke
atrasado(a) back, behind
atravesar to go through
audiencia (*f.*) (court) hearing
audífono (*m.*) hearing aid
aumentar to gain, to increase
aun even
ausente absent
auto(móvil) (*m.*) auto, car
autoridad (*f.*) authority
autorización (*f.*) authorization

autorizar to authorize
auxiliar de enfermera (*m., f.*) nurse's aide
avenida (*f.*) avenue
aventado(a) bloated
averiguar to find out
avisar to advise, to warn, to let (someone) know
aviso (*m.*) warning
¡ay! oh!
¡Ay, Dios mío! Oh, God!, Oh, my goodness!
ayer yesterday
ayuda (*f.*) help, aid
  — a familias con niños (*f.*) Aid to Families with Dependent Children (AFDC)
  — en dinero (*f.*) financial assistance
ayudar to help
ayunas: en — on an empty stomach, fasting, before eating anything
azúcar (*m.* or *f.*) sugar
azul blue

B

babero (*m.*) (baby's) bib
babuchas (*f. pl.*) slippers
bajar to go down
  — de peso to lose weight
bajo(a) low, short, under
  de bajos ingresos (*adj.*) low income
bala: herida de — (*f.*) gunshot wound
balanceado(a) balanced
bancarrota (*f.*) bankruptcy
banco (*m.*) bank
  — de sangre (*m.*) blood bank
bañadera (*f.*) bathtub

bañar(se) to bathe
bañera (*f.*) bathtub (*Puerto Rico*)
baño (*m.*) bathroom
  — de esponja (*m.*) sponge bath
barato(a) inexpensive, cheap
barbilla (*f.*) chin
barbitúrico (*m.*) barbiturate
barriga (*f.*) abdomen
barrio (*m.*) neighborhood
básico(a) basic
bastón (*m.*) cane
bata (*f.*) robe
batería (*f.*) battery
bazo (*m.*) spleen
bebé (*m., f.*) baby
  — de probeta (*m.*) test-tube baby
beber to drink
bebida (*f.*) beverage, drink
  — alcohólica (*f.*) alcoholic beverage
bebito (*m.*) baby
beca (*f.*) scholarship
beneficio (*m.*) benefit
biberón (*m.*) baby bottle
bien fine, well
  —, gracias. ¿Y usted? Fine, thank you. And you?
  (No) Muy —. (Not) Very well.
  Muy —, gracias. Very well, thank you.
bienes raíces (bienes inmuebles) (*m. pl.*) real estate
bilingüe bilingual
biopsia (*f.*) biopsy
bizco(a) cross-eyed
blanco(a) white

blando(a) bland (diet); soft
blanquillo (*m.*) egg (*Méx.*)
blusa (*f.*) blouse
bobo (*m.*) pacifier (*Puerto Rico*)
boca (*f.*) mouth
— **abajo** face down
— **arriba** face up
bocio (*m.*) goiter
bofetada (*f.*) slap
bolita (*f.*) little ball, lump
bolsa (*f.*) bag; handbag, purse
— **de agua** (*f.*) water bag
— **de hielo** (*f.*) ice pack
bomberos: departamento de — (*m.*) fire department
bonito(a) pretty
bono (*m.*) bond
borroso(a) blurry
botánica (*f.*) store that sells herbal medicine
botella (*f.*) bottle
botica (*f.*) pharmacy, drugstore
botiquín (*m.*) medicine chest, medicine cabinet
— **de primeros auxilios** (*m.*) first-aid kit
botón (*m.*) button
brazo (*m.*) arm
breve brief, short
brindar to offer
bróculi (*m.*) broccoli
broncoscopia, broncoscopía (*f.*) bronchoscopy
bronquitis (*f.*) bronchitis
bucal oral (*ref. to the mouth*)
bueno(a) okay, fine, well, good
buena suerte good luck
Buenas noches. Good evening., Good night.

Buenas tardes. Good afternoon.
Buenos días. Good morning., Good day.
bufanda (*f.*) scarf
buscar to look for

C

cabello (*m.*) hair
cabeza (*f.*) head
— **de familia** (*m., f.*) head of household
caca (*coll.*) (*f.*) excrement, stool
cachete (*m.*) cheek
cada every, each
— **... horas** every . . . hours
cadera (*f.*) hip
caer(se) to fall; to fall down
café (*m.*) coffee
cafeína (*f.*) caffeine
caja (*f.*) box
— **de seguridad** (*f.*) safe
— **fuerte** (*f.*) safe
cajero(a) (*m., f.*) cashier
cajetilla (*f.*) pack (*of cigarettes*)
calambre (*m.*) cramp
calcáneo (*m.*) calcaneus
calcetín (*m.*) sock
calcetines (*m. pl.*) socks
calcio (*m.*) calcium
cálculos (*m. pl.*) stones
— **en la vejiga** (*m. pl.*) bladder stones
— **en la vesícula** (*m. pl.*) gallstones
calefacción (*f.*) heat, heating
calentador (*m.*) heater
calentar (e:ie) to heat up

calentón (*m.*) heater (*Méx.*)
calentura (*f.*) fever
caliente hot
calificar to qualify
calle (*f.*) street
calmante (*m.*) painkiller, sedative
calmar(se) to calm down, to relax
caloría (*f.*) calorie
cama (*f.*) bed
cambiar to change
  — **de trabajo** to change jobs
  — **un cheque** to cash a check
cambiar(se) to change (oneself)
cambio (*m.*) change
camilla (*f.*) gurney, stretcher
caminar to walk
camioncito (*m.*) small truck
camisa (*f.*) shirt
camiseta (*f.*) T-shirt
camisón (*m.*) nightgown
campanilla (*f.*) uvula
campo (*m.*) field, country
canal (*m.*) canal
  — **auditivo** (*m.*) ear canal
  — **de la orina** (*m.*) urethra
  — **en la raíz** (*m.*) root canal
cáncer (*m.*) cancer
canino (*m.*) canine (tooth)
cansado(a) tired
cansancio (*m.*) tiredness, exhaustion, fatigue
cantidad (*f.*) amount, quantity
  — **fija** (*f.*) fixed amount
caño de la orina (*m.*) urethra
capacitación (*f.*) training

capacitado(a) able
capa de agua (*f.*) raincoat
capítulo (*m.*) chapter
cápsula (*f.*) capsule
cara (*f.*) face
caramelo (*m.*) candy
carbohidrato (*m.*) carbohydrate
cárcel (*f.*) jail
cardenal (*m.*) bruise (*Cuba*)
cardiograma (*m.*) cardiogram
cardiología (*f.*) cardiology
cardiólogo(a) cardiologist
carga (*f.*) burden
cargo (*m.*) position
cariado(a) decayed, carious
caries (*f.*) cavity
carne (*f.*) meat
caro(a) expensive
carpo (*m.*) carpus
carro (*m.*) car
carta (*f.*) letter
cartera (*f.*) handbag, purse
casa (*f.*) house, home
— **de Primeros Auxilios** (*f.*) House of First Aid
— **de Socorro** (*f.*) House of Help
— **para ancianos** (*f.*) home for the elderly
— **rodante** (*f.*) mobile home
casado(a) married
casarse (con) to marry, to get married (to)
casi almost
— **nunca** hardly ever
caso (*m.*) case
en ese — in that case

castigar to punish
cataratas (*f. pl.*) cataracts
catarro (*m.*) cold
católico(a) Catholic
causar to cause
ceguera (*f.*) blindness
ceja (*f.*) eyebrow
cemento (*m.*) cement
cena (*f.*) dinner, supper
centavo (*m.*) cent
centro (*m.*) center, downtown area
— **de cuidado de niños** (*m.*) nursery school (*Puerto Rico*)
— **de envenenamiento** (*m.*) poison center
cepillar(se) to brush (oneself)
— **los dientes** to brush one's teeth
cepillo (*m.*) brush
— **de dientes** (*m.*) toothbrush
cerca (de) close, near
cercano(a) near
cereal (*m.*) cereal
cerebro (*m.*) brain, cerebrum
cerilla (*f.*) match
cerrado(a) closed
cerrar (e:ie) to close
certificado (*m.*) certificate
— **de bautismo** (*m.*) baptismal certificate
— **de defunción** (*m.*) death certificate
— **de depósito** (*m.*) certificate of deposit (CD)
— **de matrimonio** (*m.*) marriage certificate
— **de nacimiento** (*m.*) birth certificate
cerveza (*f.*) beer
cérvix (*f.*) cervix

cesantear to fire (from a job)
cesáreo(a) cesarean
chamarra (*f.*) jacket (*Méx.*)
chancro (*m.*) chancre
chaqueta (*f.*) jacket
chata (*f.*) bedpan
chau bye
chavo (*m.*) cent (*Puerto Rico*)
cheque (*m.*) check
chequear to check
chequeo (*m.*) checkup, exam, examination
chequera (*f.*) checkbook (*Cuba y Puerto Rico*)
chicos (*m. pl.*) children
chichón (*m.*) bump (*on the head*)
chile (*m.*) pepper
chocar to run into, to collide
chocolate (*m.*) chocolate
chupete (*m.*) pacifier
chupón (*m.*) pacifier (*Méx.*)
cicatriz (*f.*) scar
ciego(a) blind
cien(to) por ciento one hundred percent
cierto(a) certain
cigarrillo (*m.*) cigarette
cinta adhesiva (*f.*) adhesive tape
cinto (*m.*) belt
cintura (*f.*) waist
cinturón (*m.*) belt
circulación (*f.*) circulation
cirugía (*f.*) surgery
cirujano(a) (*m., f.*) surgeon
cita (*f.*) appointment
ciudad (*f.*) city
ciudadanía (*f.*) citizenship

ciudadano(a) (*m., f.*) citizen
clamidia (*f.*) chlamydia
claramente clearly
claro of course
clase (*f.*) class
clavícula (*f.*) clavicle
cliente(a) (*m., f.*) client
clínica (*f.*) clinic; hospital
clínico (*m., f.*) general practitioner, internist
clínico(a) (*adj.*) medical
coágulo (*m.*) coagulum, coagulation, clot
cobija (*f.*) blanket
cobrar to charge, to get paid
  — un cheque to cash a check
coca (*f.*) cocaine
  — cocinada (*f.*) crack (*coll.*)
cocaína (*f.*) cocaine
cóccix (*m.*) coccyx
coche (*m.*) car
cochecito (*m.*) baby carriage
cocina (*f.*) kitchen, stove
cocinar to cook
cocinero(a) (*m., f.*) cook
codeína (*f.*) codeine
código postal (*m.*) zip code, postal code (*Méx.*)
codo (*m.*) elbow
coger to take
cognado (*m.*) cognate
cojo(a) one-legged; lame
col (*f.*) cabbage
colesterol (*m.*) cholesterol
cólico (*m.*) colic
colitis (*f.*) colitis
colmillo (*m.*) canine (tooth)

colocar to place
colon (*m.*) colon
colonoscopia, colonoscopía (*f.*) colonoscopy, coloscopy
columna vertebral (*f.*) backbone, spinal column
comadrona (*f.*) midwife
combustible (*m.*) fuel
comedor (*m.*) dining room
comenzar (e:ie) to begin, to start
comer to eat
comercial commercial
cometer to commit; to perpetrate
comezón (*f.*) itching
comida (*f.*) meal, food, lunch; midday meal
comidita de bebé (*f.*) baby food
comisión (*f.*) commission
como as, like, since
¿cómo? how?
 ¿— está usted? How are you?
 — no of course, sure
 ¿— se escribe... ? How do you spell . . . ?
cómoda (*f.*) chest of drawers
comodidad (*f.*) convenience
cómodo(a) comfortable
compañero(a) (*m., f.*) companion, pal, buddy
 — sexual (*m., f.*) sexual partner
compañía (*f.*) company
 — de seguro (*f.*) insurance company
comparar to compare
compartir to share
compasión (*f.*) compassion
compensación obrera (*f.*) worker's compensation
completamente completely

completar to complete
completo(a) complete
complicación (*f.*) complication
comportarse to behave
comprar to buy
comprender to understand
compresa (*f.*) compress
comprobante (*m.*) receipt
común common
con with
— **ella** with her
— **frecuencia** frequently
¿— qué frecuencia? How frequently?, How often?
concebir (e:i) to conceive
conceder un crédito to extend credit
concubinato (*m.*) common-law marriage
condado (*m.*) county
condimentado(a) spiced, spicy
condón (*m.*) condom
conducir to drive
conducto: — lacrimal (lagrimal) (*m.*) tear duct
— **auditivo** (*m.*) ear canal
confidencial confidential
confirmar to confirm
conjuntivitis (*f.*) conjunctivitis
conmigo with me
conocer to know, to be acquainted with (*a person, a place*)
conocimiento (*m.*) knowledge
perder (e:ie) el — to be unconscious, to lose consciousness
consecutivo(a) consecutive
conseguir (e:i) to get, to obtain

consejero(a) (*m., f.*) counselor
— **familiar** (*m., f.*) family counselor
consejo (*m.*) advice
consentimiento (*m.*) consent
consistir (en) to consist (of)
constantemente constantly
consultar to consult
consultorio (*m.*) doctor's office
consumir to consume
contacto (*m.*) contact
contagiar to infect
contagioso(a) contagious
contar (o:ue) to count, to tell
contener to contain
conteo (*m.*) blood count, count
contestación (*f.*) answer
contestar to answer
continuar to continue
contra against
contracción (*f.*) contraction
contraceptivo (*m.*) contraceptive
contribuyente (*m., f.*) taxpayer
control (*m.*) control
controlar to control
convaleciente (*m., f.*) convalescent
convencer to convince
conveniencia (*f.*) convenience
conversación (*f.*) conversation
conversar to talk
convertirse (e:ie) en to change into, to become
convulsiones (*f. pl.*) convulsions
cooperar to cooperate
coordinador(a) (*m., f.*) coordinator
copia (*f.*) copy

— **fotostática** (*f.*) photocopy
corazón (*m.*) heart
cordal (*m.*) wisdom tooth
cordón umbilical (*m.*) umbilical cord
corona (*f.*) crown
correctamente correctly
correcto(a) correct
correr to run
cortada (*f.*) cut (*Méx. y Cuba*)
cortadura (*f.*) cut
cortar(se) to cut (oneself)
corto(a) de vista nearsighted
cosa (*f.*) thing
cosmético(s) (*m. pl.*) cosmetics
costado (*m.*) side
costar (o:ue) to cost
costilla (*f.*) rib
costo (*m.*) cost
costra (*f.*) scab
crac (*m.*) crack
cráneo (*m.*) skull
creer to believe, to think
Creo que no. I don't think so.
Creo que sí. I think so.
crema (*f.*) cream
crianza (*f.*) raising, upbringing
criarse to be raised
crimen (*m.*) crime
crisis (*f.*) crisis
crup (*m.*) croup
cruz (*f.*) cross; X
— **Roja** (*f.*) Red Cross
cuadra (*f.*) (city) block
cuadrado (*m.*) box; square

cuadro (*m.*) box; square
¿cuál? what?, which?
cualquier(a) any
cuando when
¿cuándo? when?
cuanto antes as soon as possible
— **mejor** the sooner, the better
¿cuánto? how much?; **¿cuánto(a)?** (*adj.*) how much?
¿— mide (Ud.)? How tall are you?
¿— paga de alquiler? How much do you pay in rent?
¿— tiempo? how long?
¿— tiempo hace que... ? How long have . . . ?
¿— tiempo hace... ? How long ago. . .?
¿— tiempo hacía que... ? How long had . . . ?
¿por — tiempo... ? for how long. . .?
¿cuántos(as)? how many?
¿Cuántos años tiene Ud.? How old are you?
cuarto (*m.*) bedroom, room; quarter
— **de hora** (*m.*) quarter of an hour
cuates (*m., f. pl.*) twins (*Méx.*)
cubierto(a) covered
cúbito (*m.*) ulna
cubrir to cover
cucaracha (*f.*) cockroach; joint (*coll., drugs*)
cucharada (*f.*) (table)spoonful
cucharadita (*f.*) teaspoonful
cuello (*m.*) neck
cuenta (*f.*) bill, account
— **corriente** (*f.*) checking account
— **de ahorros** (*f.*) savings account
— **de cheques** (*f.*) checking account

cuero cabelludo (*m.*) scalp
cuerpo (*m.*) body
cuestionario (*m.*) questionnaire
cuidado (*m.*) care
cuidar to take care of
cuidar(se) to take care (of oneself)
cultural cultural
cuna (*f.*) crib, cradle
cuña (*f.*) bedpan
cuñado(a) (*m., f.*) brother-in law, sister-in-law
cupón (*m.*) coupon
— **para comida** (*m.*) food stamp
cura (*f.*) cure; (*m.*) (Catholic) priest
curado(a) cured
curandero(a) (*m., f.*) folk healer, natural healer
curar to cure
curita (*f.*) adhesive bandage, band-aid
curso (*m.*) course, class
custodia (*f.*) custody
cutis (*m.*) skin (facial)
cuyo(a) whose

D

daltonismo (*m.*) color blindness
daño (*m.*) damage
dar to give
— **a luz** to give birth
— **de alta** to release (*from a hospital*)
— **de comer** to feed, to nurse
— **de mamar** to nurse
— **el pecho** to feed, to nurse
— **golpes** to hit, to strike
— **resultado** to work, to produce results

— **una puñalada** to stab
— **un tiro** to shoot
— **viaje** to take drugs
darle vergüenza a uno to be embarrassed
darse vuelta to turn over
datos (*m. pl.*) information, data
de of
— **acuerdo con** according to
— **al lado** from next door
— **la mano** by the hand
— **la mañana (tarde, noche)** in the morning (afternoon, evening)
— **lado** on (one's) side
— **modo que** so that
— **nada.** You're welcome.
— **nuevo** again
— **prisa** in a hurry
— **rutina** routinely
— **todos modos** anyway
¿— **veras?** Really?
debajo de under
deber must, should; to owe
— **(+ *inf.*)** should (do something), must (do something)
débil weak
debilidad (*f.*) weakness
decidir to decide
decir (e:i) to say, to tell
decisión (*f.*) decision
dedo (*m.*) finger
— **del pie** (*m.*) toe
— **gordo** (*m.*) big toe
deducciones permitidas (*f. pl.*) allowable deductions

deducible deductible
defecar to have a bowel movement
defecto físico (*m.*) disability
deformar to deform
dejar to leave (behind), to let, to allow
  — de (+ *inf.*) to stop (doing something)
delgado(a) thin
delincuente juvenil (*m.*) juvenile delinquent
delírium tremens (*m. pl.*) DT's
delito (*m.*) crime; felony, misdemeanor; transgression of law
demanda (*f.*) lawsuit
demandar to sue
demás: los (las) — (*m., f.*) (the) others
demasiado too much
demorar to take (time)
denegado(a) denied
dentadura (*f.*) teeth, set of teeth
  — postiza (*f.*) dentures
dental dental
dentina (*f.*) dentine
dentista (*m., f.*) dentist
dentro inside
  — de in, within
  por — on the inside
denuncia (*f.*) accusation, report (of a crime)
denunciar to report (a crime), to accuse
departamento (*m.*) department
  — de Bienestar Social (*m.*) Social Welfare Department
  — de Protección de Niños (*m.*) Children's Protection Department
  — de Sanidad (*m.*) Health Department
depender to depend

dependiente (*m., f.*) dependent
depósito de seguridad (*m.*) security deposit
depresión (*f.*) depression
— **nerviosa** (*f.*) nervous depression
derecha (*f.*) right (direction)
derecho (*m.*) right (law)
— **a visitar** (*m.*) visitation rights
derecho(a) right
dermatólogo(a) (*m., f.*) dermatologist
derrame (*m.*) stroke
— **cerebral** (*m.*) stroke
desalojado(a) homeless
desalojar to vacate
desalojo (*m.*) eviction
desarrollar to develop
desayuno (*m.*) breakfast
descansar to rest
descomponerse to break
descompuesto(a) out of order, broken down
descongestionantes (*m. pl.*) decongestants
descontar (o:ue) to deduct
descubrir to discover
descuento (*m.*) discount
descuidar to neglect
desde since, from
desear to wish, to want
desgraciadamente unfortunately
desinfectar to disinfect
desintoxicación (*f.*) detoxification
desmayarse to faint, to lose consciousness
desocupado(a) jobless; vacant
desocupar to vacate
despacio slowly
despedida (*f.*) farewell

despedir (e:i) to fire from a job
despertar (e:ie) to wake (someone) up
despertarse (e:ie) to wake up
despierto(a) awake
desprendimiento (*m.*) detachment
después (de) after, afterward, later
desquitar(se) to get even with
destruir to destroy
detener to stop, to arrest
detergente (*m.*) detergent
determinar to determine
deuda (*f.*) debt
día (*m.*) day
  — de fiesta (*m.*) holiday
  — feriado (*m.*) holiday
diabetes (*f.*) diabetes
diabético(a) diabetic
diafragma (*m.*) diaphragm
diagnosticar to diagnose
diagnóstico (*m.*) diagnosis
diariamente (*adv.*) daily
diario(a) (*adj.*) daily; per day
diarrea (*f.*) diarrhea
diente (*m.*) tooth
dieta (*f.*) diet
  seguir (e:i) una — to go on a diet
dietista (*m., f.*) dietician
diferente different
difícil difficult
dificultad (*f.*) difficulty
  — del habla (*f.*) speech impediment
difteria (*f.*) diphtheria
digerir (e:ie) to digest
digestivo(a) digestive

dilatado(a) dilated
dinero (*m.*) money
Dios quiera. I hope (God grant).
diploma (*m.*) diploma
dirección (*f.*) address
directamente directly, straight
director(a) (*m.*) **(de la escuela)** principal (at a school)
directorio telefónico (*m.*) telephone book
dirigir to direct
disciplina (*f.*) discipline
disciplinar to discipline
discriminación (*f.*) discrimination
discutir to discuss
disgustado(a) upset
disminuir to cut down, to diminish
disponible available
distinguir to distinguish
distinto(a) different
diurético (*m.*) diuretic
dividendo (*m.*) dividend
divorciado(a) divorced
divorciarse to divorce
doblar to bend
doctor(a) (*m., f.*) doctor
documento (*m.*) document
dólar (*m.*) dollar
doler (o:ue) to hurt, to ache
dolor (*m.*) pain, ache
  — de cabeza (*m.*) headache
  — de estómago (*m.*) stomachache
  — de garganta (*m.*) sore throat
  — de parto (*m.*) labor pain
  El — se me pasa. The pain goes away.

doloroso(a) painful
domicilio (*m.*) address
donante (*m., f.*) donor
donar to donate
¿dónde? where?
dormido(a) asleep
dormir (o:ue) to sleep
dormitorio (*m.*) bedroom
dosis (*f.*) dosage
drenaje (*m.*) drainage
droga (*f.*) drug
drogadicto(a) (*m., f.*) drug addict
droguería (*f.*) pharmacy (*coll. in some L.A. countries*)
droguero(a) (*m., f.*) person who uses or sells illicit drugs
dudar to doubt
dueño(a) de la casa (*m., f.*) landlord, landlady
dulce (*m.*) candy, sweet
durante during
durar to last
durazno (*m.*) peach
duro(a) hard, difficult

E

eccema (*m.*) eczema
económico(a) financial
eczema (*m.*) eczema
edad (*f.*) age
efectivo(a) effective
efecto (*m.*) effect
— **secundario** (*m.*) side effect
eficaz effective

ejemplo (*m.*) example
ejercicio (*m.*) exercise
el (la) que the one who
elástico(a) elastic
electricidad (*f.*) electricity
eléctrico(a) electric, electrical
electrocardiograma (*m.*) electrocardiogram (EKG)
electrodoméstico (*m.*) electrical (household) appliance
electroencefalograma (*m.*) electroencephalogram (EEG)
elegibilidad (*f.*) eligibility
elegible eligible
elegir (e:i) to choose, to select
elevado(a) elevated
elevador (*m.*) elevator
eliminar to eliminate
embarazada pregnant
embarazo (*m.*) pregnancy
embolia (*f.*) blood clot, embolism, clot, stroke
emborracharse to get drunk
emergencia (*f.*) emergency
empastar to fill (*a tooth*)
empeorar to get worse
empezar (e:ie) to begin, to start
empleado(a) (*m., f.*) employee, clerk
empleador (*m.*) employer
emplear to employ
empleo (*m.*) job
emplomar to fill (*a tooth*)
empujar to push
en at, in
— **ayunas** fasting, with an empty stomach

— **casa** at home
— **caso de** in case of
— **cuanto** as soon as
— **efectivo** in cash
— **ese caso** in that case
— **estas situaciones** in these situations
— **este momento** at the moment
— **estos días** these days
¿— **qué puedo ayudarle?** What can I do for you?
¿— **qué puedo servirle?** How may I help you?
— **seguida** right away
— **uso** in use
encargarse (de) to be in charge (of)
enchufe (*m.*) electrical outlet, socket
— **de seguridad** (*m.*) electrical plug cover
encías (*f. pl.*) gums
encinta pregnant
encontrar (o:ue) to find
endocrinólogo(a) (*m., f.*) endocrinologist
endometrosis, endometriosis (*f.*) endometriosis
endoscopia, endoscopía (*f.*) endoscopy
endrogarse to take drugs, to become addicted to drugs
endulzado(a) sweetened
endurecimiento (*m.*) hardening
enema (*m.*) enema
enfermarse to get sick, to fall ill
enfermedad (*f.*) sickness, disease
enfermero(a) (*m., f.*) nurse
— **visitador(a)** (*m., f.*) visiting nurse
enfermo(a) (*m., f.*) ill, sick, sick person

enganche (*m.*) down payment (*Méx.*)
enfisema (*m.*) emphysema
enjuagar(se) to rinse (out)
enjuague (*m.*) mouthwash
enojado(a) angry
enterarse de to find out about
entonces then
entrada (*f.*) down payment; entrance, entry; income; opening
— **bruta** (*f.*) gross earnings
— **neta** (*f.*) net income
entrante next
entrar (en) to enter; to go (come) in
entre between, among
entregar to deliver
entrenamiento (*m.*) training
entrevista (*f.*) interview
entrevistar to interview
entumecido(a) numb
entumecimiento (*m.*) numbness
envenenamiento (*m.*) poisoning
envenenar(se) to poison (oneself)
enviar to send
enyesar to put a cast on
epidemia (*f.*) epidemic
epilepsia (*f.*) epilepsy
equipo (*m.*) equipment
— **electrodoméstico** (*m.*) electrical (household) appliance
equis (*f.*) cross; X
eructar to burp
erupción (*f.*) rash
Es cierto. That's right., It's true.
Es decir... That is to say . . .

escalera (*f.*) stairs, staircase
escalofríos (*m. pl.*) chills
escanograma (*m.*) CAT scan
escayola (*f.*) cast (*España*)
escayolar to put a cast on (*España*)
esclerosis múltiple (*f.*) multiple sclerosis
escoger to choose
escribir to write
— **a máquina** to type
escrito(a) written
escritorio (*m.*) desk
escroto (*m.*) scrotum
escuela (*f.*) school
— **nocturna** (*f.*) night school
— **secundaria** (*f.*) secondary school (junior and high school)
escupir to spit
escusado (*m.*) bathroom (*Méx.*)
ese(a) that
esencial essential
esmalte (*m.*) enamel
eso that
— **es todo**. That's all.
por — that's why, for that reason
espacio (*m.*) room, space
— **en blanco** (*m.*) blank space
espaguetis (*m. pl.*) spaghetti
espalda (*f.*) back
español (*m.*) Spanish (language)
esparadrapo (*m.*) adhesive bandage
especial special
especialista (*m., f.*) specialist
especialmente especially
especificar to specify

espejuelos (*m. pl.*) eyeglasses (*Cuba y Puerto Rico*)
esperar to wait (for); to hope
esperma (*f.*) sperm
espina dorsal (*f.*) spinal column
espinal spinal
espinilla (*f.*) blackhead
esponja (*f.*) sponge
esposo(a) (*m., f.*) husband, wife
espuma (*f.*) foam
esputo (*m.*) sputum
esqueleto (*m.*) skeleton
esquina (*f.*) corner
esquizofrenia (*f.*) schizophrenia
Está bien. Okay., That's fine.
esta noche tonight
estacionamiento (*m.*) parking
estado (*m.*) state, status
— **civil** (*m.*) marital status
estampilla para alimento (*f.*) food stamp
estante (*m.*) bookcase
estar to be
— **acatarrado(a)** to have a cold
— **bien** to be well, okay
— **de acuerdo** to agree
— **de parto** to be in labor
— **enfermo(a) del corazón** to have heart problems
— **en libertad bajo fianza** to be free on bail
— **en libertad condicional** to be on probation
— **resfriado(a)** to have a cold
— **equivocado(a)** to be wrong
— **preso(a)** to be in jail

— **sin trabajo** to be unemployed (out of work)
estatal (*adj.*) state
este(a) this
éste(a) (*m., f.*) this one
esterilidad (*f.*) sterility
esterilizar to sterilize
esternón (*m.*) sternum
esteroides anabólicos (*m. pl.*) anabolic steroids
estimado (*m.*) estimate
estómago (*m.*) stomach
estos(as) these
estrecho(a) narrow
estreñido(a) constipated
estrés (*m.*) stress
estricto(a) strict
estuche (de primeros auxilios) (*m.*) first-aid kit
estudiar to study
estufa (*f.*) heater; stove
evacuar to have a bowel movement (*Méx.*)
evitar to avoid
ex former
examen (*m.*) exam, examination, checkup
— **de la vista** (*m.*) eye examination
— **del oído** (*m.*) hearing test
examinar to examine
exceso de peso (*m.*) overweight
excremento (*m.*) excrement
excusado (*m.*) bathroom
exento(a) exempt
expectorar to expectorate
expediente médico (*m.*) patient's medical record

explicar to explain
exponer(se) to expose oneself
expresión (*f.*) expression
éxtasis (*m.*) ecstasy
extender (e:ie) to stretch, to extend
extra extra
extracción (*f.*) extraction
extraer to extract, to take (pull) out
extranjero(a) (*m., f.*) foreigner; (*adj.*) foreign
extraño(a) strange, unknown
extremidad (*f.*) limb
eyacular to ejaculate

F

fábrica (*f.*) factory
fácil easy
factoría (*f.*) factory
falange (*f.*) phalange
falda (*f.*) skirt
fallecido(a) deceased
faltar a clase to miss class
faltarle algo a uno to be lacking something
familia (*f.*) family
familiar family (*adj.*)
farfallotas (*f. pl.*) mumps (*Puerto Rico*)
farmacia (*f.*) pharmacy, drugstore
favor (*m.*) favor
 — de (+ *inf.*) please (do something)
fe de bautismo (*f.*) baptism certificate
fecha (*f.*) date
 — de hoy (*f.*) today's date
 — de nacimiento (*f.*) date of birth
federal federal

fémur (*m.*) femur
fértil fertile
feto (*m.*) fetus
fianza (*f.*) bail
fibra (*f.*) fiber
fíbula (*f.*) fibula
fiebre (*f.*) fever
— **del heno** (*f.*) hay fever
— **escarlatina** (*f.*) scarlet fever
— **reumática** (*f.*) rheumatic fever
fielmente faithfully
fijo(a) fixed
fin de semana (*m.*) weekend
final (*m.*) end
finalmente finally
finanzas (*f. pl.*) finance
firma (*f.*) signature
firmar to sign
físico(a) physical
flato (*m.*) intestinal gas
flema (*f.*) phlegm
flujo (*m.*) discharge
fluoroscopia, fluoroscopía (*f.*) fluoroscopy
fluoruro (*m.*) fluoride
fogón (*m.*) stove
folleto (*m.*) brochure, pamphlet
fondo mutuo (*m.*) mutual fund
fórceps (*m. sing., pl.*) forceps
forma (*f.*) form (*Méx.*); way
fórmula (*f.*) formula
forzar (o:ue) to force
fósforo (*m.*) match
fotocopia (*f.*) photocopy
fotografía (*f.*) photograph

fractura (*f.*) fracture
fracturar(se) to break, to fracture
frasco (*m.*) bottle
frazada (*f.*) blanket
frecuencia (*f.*) frequency
  con — frequently
  ¿Con qué —? How frequently?
frecuente frequent
frecuentemente frequently
frenos (*m. pl.*) dental braces
frente (*f.*) forehead
fresa (*f.*) strawberry
fricción (*f.*) rub, rubbing, massage
frijoles (*m. pl.*) beans
frío(a) cold
frustrado(a) frustrated
fuente (*f.*) source
  — de agua water bag
fuente de ingreso (*f.*) source of income
fuera outside
  — de lo común out of the ordinary
  — del alcance out of reach
  por — on the outside
fuerte strong
fumar to smoke

G

gafas (*f. pl.*) glasses
galleta (*f.*) slap (*Cuba y Puerto Rico*)
galletica (*f.*) cookie
ganancia (*f.*) gain; earning, profit
ganar to earn, to gain
ganglio linfático (*m.*) lymph gland

garaje (*m.*) garage
garganta (*f.*) throat
garrotillo (*m.*) croup
gas (*m.*) gas
gasa (*f.*) gauze
gasolina (*f.*) gasoline
gastar to spend (money)
gasto (*m.*) expense
— **de la casa** (*m.*) household expense
— **de transportación** (*m.*) transportation expense
— **funerario** (*m.*) funeral expense
gastritis (*f.*) gastritis
gatear to crawl
gemelos(as) (*m., f. pl.*) twins
general general
generalmente generally
genitales (*m. pl.*) genitals
gente (*f.*) people
geriatra (*m., f.*) geriatrician, geriatrist
ginecología (*f.*) gynecology
ginecólogo(a) (*m., f.*) gynecologist
glande (*m.*) glans
glándula (*f.*) gland
glaucoma (*m.*) glaucoma
globo (*m.*) balloon (*coll., drug dosage*)
glúteos (*m. pl.*) buttocks
golpear to hit, to strike
golpear(se) to hit (oneself)
gonorrea (*f.*) gonorrhea
gordo(a) fat
gordura (*f.*) obesity
gorro (*m.*) bonnet, cap
gota (*f.*) drop

gotero (*m.*) eyedropper
gracias thank you
Muchas —. Thank you very much.
grado (*m.*) degree
grande big, large
grano (*m.*) pimple
grasa (*f.*) fat
grasiento(a) oily
gratis (*adv.*) free (of charge), without cost
gratuito(a) (*adj.*) free (of charge)
grave serious
gripa (*f.*) flu (*Méx.*)
gripe (*f.*) flu, influenza
grupo (*m.*) group
guantes (*m. pl.*) gloves
guardado(a) put away
guardar to put away, to keep, to save
guardería (*f.*) nursery school
guía (*f.*) guide
— telefónica (*f.*) telephone book
gustar to be pleasing to, to like
gusto (*m.*) pleasure

H

haber to have
— trabajado to have worked
había there was, there were
habichuelas (*f. pl.*) beans (*Puerto Rico*)
habitación (*f.*) bedroom, room
hablar to speak, to talk
hace como... about . . .
hace un mes a month ago

hacer to do, to make
  — **caca** to have a bowel movement (*coll.*)
  — **daño** to hurt
  — **ejercicio** to exercise
  — **falta** to need
  — **gárgaras** to gargle
  — **la comida** to cook (prepare) dinner
  — **preguntas** to ask questions
  — **saber** to advise, to warn, to let (someone) know
  — **un análisis** to run a test
  — **un examen** to give a checkup
  — **una declaración falsa** to make a false statement
  — **una prueba** to run a test
hacerse to become
hachich (hashís) (*m.*) hashish
hacia toward
  — **abajo** down, downward
  — **adelante** forward
  — **atrás** backwards
hágame el favor de (+ *inf.*) Please (+ *command*)
hambre: tener — to be hungry
hamburguesa (*f.*) hamburger
harina (*f.*) flour
hasta until, till
  — **hace poco** until recently
  — **luego.** See you later.
  — **mañana.** See you tomorrow.
  — **que** until
hay there is, there are
  No — de qué. You're welcome.
helado(a) ice, iced

hemorragia (*f.*) hemorrhage
— **cerebral** (*f.*) stroke
hemorroide (*f.*) hemorroid
hepatitis (*f.*) hepatitis
hereditario(a) hereditary
herencia (*f.*) inheritance
herida (*f.*) wound, injury
herido(a) (*m., f.*) injured person
hermanastro(a) (*m., f.*) stepbrother; stepsister
hermano(a) (*m., f.*) brother, sister
heroína (*f.*) heroin
herpes (*m. sing.*) herpes
hidropesía (*f.*) dropsy
hielo (*m.*) ice
hierro (*m.*) iron
hígado (*m.*) liver
higienista (*m., f.*) hygienist
hijastro(a) stepson, stepdaughter
hijo(a) (*m., f.*) son, daughter
— **de crianza** (*m., f.*) foster child
hijos (*m. pl.*) children
hinchazón (*f.*) bump, swelling
hiperopía (*f.*) farsightedness
hipertensión (*f.*) hypertension, high blood pressure
hipoteca (*f.*) mortgage
hirviendo boiling
histerectomía (*f.*) hysterectomy
historia clínica (*f.*) medical history
hogar (*m.*) home
— **de crianza** (*m.*) foster home
— **sustituto** (*m.*) foster home
hoja (*f.*) sheet (of paper)
— **clínica** (*f.*) medical history

hola hello
hombre (*m.*) man
hombro (*m.*) shoulder
hondo deep (*adv.*); deep (*adj.*)
hongo (*m.*) fungus
honorario de corredor (*m.*) broker's fee
hora (*f.*) hour
 — de visita (*f.*) visiting hour
horario (*m.*) hours, schedule
hormigueo (*m.*) pins and needles, tingling
horno (*m.*) oven
hospital (*m.*) hospital
hospitalización (*f.*) hospitalization
hospitalizado(a) hospitalized
hotel (*m.*) hotel
hoy today
 — mismo this very day
hueco (*m.*) hole
huelga (*f.*) strike
hueso (*m.*) bone
 — ilíaco (*m.*) ilium
huevo (*m.*) egg
humano(a) human
húmero (*m.*) humerus

I

idea (*f.*) idea
identificación (*f.*) identification
idioma (*m.*) language
iglesia (*f.*) church
ilegal illegal
indocumentado(a) undocumented (*without immigration papers*)

immunodeficiencia (*f.*) immunodeficiency
impermeable (*m.*) raincoat
implante (*m.*) implant
imponer una multa to give a fine (ticket)
importancia (*f.*) importance
importante important
importar to matter
A nadie le importa. It's nobody's business.
No importa. It doesn't matter.
imposible impossible
impotencia (*f.*) impotence
impuesto (*m.*) tax
— **sobre la propiedad** (*m.*) property tax
— **sobre la renta** (*m.*) income tax
incapacidad (*f.*) disability
incapacitado(a) incapacitated, handicapped
— **para trabajar** unable to work
incendio (*m.*) fire
incesto (*m.*) incest
incisivo (*m.*) incisor
incluido(a) including
incluir to include
incubación (*f.*) incubation
incubadora (*f.*) incubator
independiente independent
indicar to indicate
infarto (*m.*) heart attack
infección (*f.*) infection
— **de la garganta** (*f.*) tonsilitis
infeccioso(a) infectious
infectar to infect
inflamación (*f.*) inflamation
— **del intestino grueso** (*f.*) colitis
inflamado(a) swollen

inflamatorio(a) inflammatory
influenza (*f.*) flu
información (*f.*) information
  — sobre el caso (*f.*) case history
informar to inform, to notify
informe (*m.*) report
ingle (*f.*) groin
inglés (*m.*) English (language)
ingresar to admit (*to a hospital*), to be admitted
ingreso (*m.*) income, earnings, revenue
  de bajos ingresos low-income
inicial (*f.*) initial
iniciar to start, to initiate
inmediatamente immediately
inmigración (*f.*) immigration
inmigrante (*m., f.*) immigrant
inodoro (*m.*) toilet
inscripción (*f.*) certificate
  — de bautismo (*f.*) baptism certificate
  — de defunción (*f.*) death certificate
  — de matrimonio (*f.*) marriage certificate
  — de nacimiento (*f.*) birth certificate (*Cuba*)
insecticida (*m.*) insecticide
inseminación artificial (*f.*) artificial insemination
insertar to insert
insolación (*f.*) sunstroke
insomnio (*m.*) insomnia
insoportable unbearable
instrucción (*f.*) instruction
insulina (*f.*) insulin
intensivo(a) intensive
interés (*m.*) interest
internar to be admitted (*to a hospital*)

internista (*m., f.*) general practitioner, internist
interno(a) internal
intestino (*m.*) gut, intestine
— **delgado** (*m.*) small intestine
— **grueso** (*m.*) large intestine
intoxicación (*f.*) intoxication
inválido(a) disabled; crippled
inversión (*f.*) investment
investigador(a) (*m., f.*) investigator
investigar to investigate
invierno (*m.*) winter
inyección (*f.*) injection, shot
— **antitetánica** (*f.*) tetanus shot
— **contra el tétano** (*f.*) tetanus shot
inyectar(se) to inject (oneself)
ipecacuana (*f.*) (syrup of) ipecac
ir to go
— **a (+ *inf.*)** to be going to (do something)
— **y venir** to commute
irritación (*f.*) irritation
irritado(a) irritated
irse to leave, to go away
izquierda (*f.*) left
izquierdo(a) left

J

jabón (*m.*) soap
jalea (*f.*) jelly
jaqueca(s) (*f.*) migraine
jarabe (*m.*) syrup
— **para la tos** (*m.*) cough syrup
jardín (*m.*) garden
jardinero(a) (*m., f.*) gardener

jefe(a) (*m., f.*) boss, chief
— de familia (*m., f.*) head of household
jeringa (hipodérmica) (*f.*) hypodermic syringe
jeringuilla (*f.*) hypodermic syringe
jimaguas (*m., f. pl.*) twins (*Cuba*)
joven young
joyas (*f. pl.*) jewelry
juanete (*m.*) bunion
jubilación (*f.*) retirement
jubilado(a) retired
jubilarse to retire
judío(a) Jewish
juez(a) (*m., f.*) judge
jugar (u:ue) to play (*a game*)
— con fuego to play with fire
jugo (*m.*) juice
— de china orange juice (*Puerto Rico*)
— de naranja orange juice
juguetón(ona) mischievous, restless
junto(a) together
justo(a) fair
juzgado (*m.*) courthouse

L

la que the one who
labio (*m.*) lip
laboratorio (*m.*) laboratory
lado (*m.*) side
al — de at the side of
ladrón(ona) (*m., f.*) burglar
lámpara (*f.*) lamp
laparoscopia, laparoscopía (*f.*) laparoscopy
lápiz (*m.*) pencil

laringitis (*f.*) laryngitis
lastimar to hurt
lastimarse to get hurt, to hurt oneself
latido (*m.*) heartbeat
latir to beat (heart)
lavado (*m.*) washing
  hacer un — de estómago to pump the stomach
  — intestinal (*m.*) enema
lavativa (*f.*) enema
laxante (*m.*) laxative
leche (*f.*) milk
  — descremada (*f.*) skim milk
leer to read
legal legal
legumbre (*f.*) vegetable
lejía (*f.*) bleach
lejos (de) far away
lengua (*f.*) tongue; language
leño (*m.*) joint (*coll.*)
lentamente slowly
lentes (*m. pl.*) glasses
  — de contacto (*m. pl.*) contact lenses
lesión (*f.*) injury, lesion
letra (*f.*) handwriting, letter
  — de imprenta (*f.*) print, printed letter
  — de molde (*f.*) print, printed letter
leucemia (*f.*) leukemia
levantar(se) to lift, to raise, to get up
  al — first thing in the morning
ley (*f.*) law
libertad (*f.*) freedom
  — bajo fianza (*f.*) out on bail
  — condicional (*f.*) probation

libra (*f.*) pound
libreta de ahorros (*f.*) savings passbook
libro (*m.*) book
— **de texto** (*m.*) textbook
licencia (*f.*) license
— **de conducir** (*f.*) driver's license
— **para cuidar niños** (*f.*) child care license
ligadura (*f.*) tourniquet
ligar to tie
— **los tubos** to tie the tubes
ligero(a) light
limitación (*f.*) limitation
limitado(a) limited
limpiar to clean
limpieza (*f.*) cleaning
línea (*f.*) line; line (on a paper or form)
— **de ayuda a los padres** (*f.*) parent help line
linimento (*m.*) liniment
líquido (*m.*) liquid
lista (*f.*) list
listo(a) ready
llaga (*f.*) sore, wound
llamado(a) called
llamar to call
— **por teléfono** to phone
llamarse to be called, to be named
llegar to arrive
llenar to fill out
lleno(a) de gases bloated
llevar to take (someone or something somewhere), to carry
— **a cabo** to carry out
llevarse bien to get along well

llorar to cry
lo it, him, you (*form.*)
— **más pronto posible** as soon as possible
— **mejor** the best (thing)
— **mismo** the same (thing)
— **primero** the first thing
— **que** that which, what
— **sé.** I know.
— **siento.** I'm sorry.
— **suficiente** enough
local local
loción (*f.*) lotion
— **para bebé** (*f.*) baby lotion
locura (*f.*) insanity
lonche (*m.*) lunch (*coll., Méx.*)
los (las) demás (*m., f.*) the others
los (las) dos both, the two of them
lubricar to lubricate
luego then
lugar (*m.*) place
— **de nacimiento** (*m.*) place of birth
— **donde trabaja** (*m.*) place of employment
lunar (*m.*) mole
luz (*f.*) light

M

macarrones (*m. pl.*) macaroni
machismo (*m.*) male chauvinism
madrastra (*f.*) stepmother
madre (*f.*) mother
madurar to mature
maestro(a) (*m., f.*) teacher
majadero(a) mischievous, restless

mal badly
mal de ojo (*m.*) evil eye
malaria (*f.*) malaria
malestar (*m.*) discomfort, malaise
maligno(a) malignant
malo(a) bad
malparto (*m.*) miscarriage
maltratar to abuse, to mistreat
maltrato (*m.*) abuse
mamá (*f.*) mother, mom
mamadera (*f.*) baby bottle
mamar: dar de — to nurse
mamila (*f.*) baby bottle (*Méx.*)
mamografía (*f.*) mammogram
mancha en la piel (*f.*) birthmark
manco(a) one-handed
mandar to send
mandíbula (*f.*) jawbone
manga (*f.*) sleeve
manejar to drive
  — estando borracho(a) drunk driving
manera (*f.*) way
manifestarse (e:ie) to manifest
mano (*f.*) hand
manta (*f.*) blanket
manteca (*f.*) heroin (*coll., Caribe*)
mantener(se) (e:ie) to keep, to support (oneself)
mantequilla (*f.*) butter
  — de cacahuate (*f.*) peanut butter
  — de maní (*f.*) peanut butter
manzana (*f.*) apple
mañana (*adv.*) tomorrow; (*f.*) morning
maquillaje (*m.*) makeup
máquina (*f.*) car (*Cuba*)

maravilloso(a) wonderful
marca (*f.*) mark
marcapasos (*m. sing.*) pacemaker
marcar to mark; to check off
mareo (*m.*) dizziness
margarina (*f.*) margarine
marido (*m.*) husband
mariguana (marihuana) (*f.*) marijuana
más more, else, most
  — adelante later on
  — de (+ *número*) more than (+ *number*)
  — o menos more or less
  — ... que more . . . than
  — que nunca more than ever
  — tarde later
masa (*f.*) mass
matar to kill
matrícula (*f.*) registration
matarse to kill oneself, to commit suicide
materia fecal (*f.*) stool, feces
matricularse to register
matrimonio (*m.*) marriage
matriz (*f.*) womb
mayor major, older, oldest
  — de edad of age
  el (la) — the oldest
mayoría (*f.*) majority
mechón (*m.*) patch
media hora (*f.*) half an hour
medianoche (*f.*) midnight
  a (la) — at midnight
medias (*f. pl.*) stockings
  — de hombre (*f. pl.*) socks
  — elásticas (*f. pl.*) support stockings

medicina (*f.*) medicine
medicinal medicinal, medicated
médico(a) (*adj.*) medical; (*m., f.*) doctor, M.D.
medio(a) half
— **hermano(a)** (*m., f.*) half-brother, half-sister
medio: en el — in the middle
mediodía (*m.*) midday, noon
medir (e:i) to measure, to be . . . tall
mejilla (*f.*) cheek
mejor better, best
mejorar to make better, to improve
mejorarse to get better
mellizos(as) (*m., f. pl.*) twins
melocotón (*m.*) peach
melón (*m.*) melon
meningitis (*f.*) meningitis
menor minor, younger, youngest
el (la) — the youngest
— de edad minor
menos less, fewer
— de (+ *número*) less than (+ *number*)
— mal thank goodness
por lo — at least
—... que less . . . than
menstruación (*f.*) menstruation
mensual monthly
mental mental
mentir (e:ie) to lie, to tell a lie
mentira (*f.*) lie
mentón (*m.*) chin
mercado (*m.*) market
mes (*m.*) month
mesa (*f.*) table

mesita de noche (*f.*) night table
metadona (*f.*) methadone
metatarso (*m.*) metatarsus
meterse en la boca to put in one's mouth
método (*m.*) method
mi(s) my
miel (*f.*) honey
miembro (*m.*) member; penis
mientras while
  — tanto in the meantime
migraña (*f.*) migraine
mineral (*m.*) mineral
minuto (*m.*) minute
mío(a) mine
miope nearsighted
miopía (*f.*) nearsightedness
mirar to look at
mismo(a) same
  el (la) — que antes the same as before
mitad (*f.*) half
molar (*m.*) molar
molestia (*f.*) trouble, discomfort
molesto(a) annoyed, bothered
momento (*m.*) moment
momentico (*m.*) a short time
momentito (*m.*) a short time
moneda (*f.*) coin
monga (*f.*) influenza (*coll., Puerto Rico*)
monitorizado(a) monitored
morado (*m.*) bruise
morder (o:ue) to bite
mordida (*f.*) bite
moretón (*m.*) bruise
morfina (*f.*) morphine

morir (o:ue) to die
mover(se) (o:ue) to move
— **el vientre** to have a bowel movement
muchacho(a) (*m., f.*) boy, young man; girl, young woman
Muchas gracias. (*f. pl.*) Many thanks., Thanks a lot.
muchas veces many times
muchísimo(a) very much
mucho much, a lot
mucosas (*f. pl.*) mucous membranes
mudanza (*f.*) moving (*to another lodging*)
mudarse to move (*to another lodging*)
mudo(a) mute
mueble (*m.*) piece of furniture
muebles (*m. pl.*) furniture
muela (*f.*) molar; tooth
— **del juicio** (*f.*) wisdom tooth
muerte (*f.*) death
muestra (*f.*) sample, specimen
— **de excremento** (*f.*) stool specimen
— **de heces fecales** (*f.*) stool specimen
— **de orina** (*f.*) urine sample (specimen)
mujer (*f.*) wife, woman
mujercita (*f.*) female (girl) (*coll., Méx.*)
muleta (*f.*) crutch
muñeca (*f.*) wrist
músculo (*m.*) muscle
muslo (*m.*) thigh
muy very
— **amable** very kind (of you)

N

nacer to be born
nacimiento (*m.*) birth
nacionalidad (*f.*) nationality
nada nothing
  — más que just
nadie anyone, nobody, no one
nalga (*f.*) buttock, rump
nalgada (*f.*) spanking
naranja (*f.*) orange
nariz (*f.*) nose
natalidad (*f.*) birth
náusea (*f.*) nausea
Navidad (*f.*) Christmas
necesariamente necessarily
necesario(a) necessary
necesidad (*f.*) need
necesitar to need
negarse (e:ie) to refuse
negativo(a) negative
negro(a) black
nervio (*m.*) nerve
nervioso(a) nervous
neto(a) net
neumonía (*f.*) pneumonia
neurología (*f.*) neurology
neurológico(a) neurological
neurólogo(a) (*m., f*) neurologist
ni neither
  — un centavo not a cent
  —... ni neither . . . nor
nieto(a) (*m., f.*) grandson, granddaughter
ningún(a) no, not any

ninguno(a) not a one, none
niñera (*f.*) nanny
niño(a) (*m., f.*) child, boy (girl)
nitroglicerina (*f.*) nitroglycerin
no no
— **andar bien** to not go well
— **es así.** It is not that way.
— **hay de qué.** You're welcome.
— **importa.** It doesn't matter.
— **importarle a nadie** to be nobody's business
— **más que** just
noche (*f.*) night, evening
nombre (*m.*) name, noun
— **de pila** (*m.*) first name
normal normal
normalmente normally
norteamericano(a) (North) American
nosotros(as) us, we
nota (*f.*) note
notar to notice
notario(a) público(a) (*m., f.*) notary (public)
notificar to report, to notify
novio(a) (*m., f.*) boyfriend, girlfriend
novocaína (*f.*) novocaine
nuca (*f.*) nape
nudillo (*m.*) knuckle
nuera (*f.*) daughter-in-law
nuestro(a) our
nuevo(a) new
numerado(a) numbered
número (*m.*) number
— **de teléfono** (*m.*) telephone number
nunca never

O

o or
obesidad (*f.*) obesity
objeto (*m.*) object
obrar to have a bowel movement
obrero(a) (*m., f.*) worker; laborer
obstetra (*m., f.*) obstetrician
obstruido(a) clogged
obtener to get, to obtain
ocupado(a) busy
oculista (*m., f.*) oculist, ophthalmologist, optometrist
ocupación (*f.*) occupation
ocurrir to happen, to occur
odontólogo(a) (*m., f.*) odontologist; dental surgeon; dentist
oficina (*f.*) office
oficio (*m.*) trade
oftalmología (*f.*) ophthalmology
oftalmólogo(a) (*m., f.*) ophthalmologist
oído (*m.*) (inner, internal) ear
oír to hear
ojalá I hope, if only (God grant)
ojo (*m.*) eye
olor (*m.*) odor
olvidarse (de) to forget
ombligo (*m.*) navel
omóplato (*m.*) scapula
oncólogo(a) (*m., f.*) oncologist
opción (*f.*) option
operación (*f.*) operation, surgery
— **de corazón abierto** (*f.*) open heart surgery
operar to operate

operarse to have surgery
opio (*m.*) opium
opresión (*f.*) tightness
opuesto(a) opposite
orden (*f.*) order, referral
— **de detención** (*f.*) warrant; order
ordenar to order
oreja (*f.*) (external) ear
organización (*f.*) organization
órgano (*m.*) organ
original original
orina (*f.*) urine
orinar to urinate
ortodoncia (*f.*) orthodontia
ortodoncista (*m., f.*) orthodontist
ortopeda (*m., f.*) orthopedist
ortopedia (*f.*) orthopedics
ortopédico(a) orthopedic
ortopedista (*m., f.*) orthopedist
otoño (*m.*) autumn, fall
orzuelo (*m.*) sty
oscuridad (*f.*) dark, darkness
otorrinolaringólogo(a) (*m., f.*) ear, nose, and throat specialist
otra persona (*f.*) someone else
otra vez again
otro(a) other, another
el (la) — the other
ovario (*m.*) ovary
ovulación (*f.*) ovulation
óvulo (*m.*) ovum
oxígeno (*m.*) oxygen

P

paciencia (*f.*) patience
paciente (*m., f.*) patient
— **externo(a)** (*m., f.*) outpatient
— **interno(a)** (*m., f.*) inpatient
padecer to suffer
— **del corazón** to have heart trouble
padrastro (*m.*) stepfather
padre (*m.*) father, dad; (Catholic) priest
padres (*m. pl.*) parents
— **de crianza** (*m. pl.*) foster parents
pagar to pay
— **a plazos** to pay in installments
página (*f.*) page
pago (*m.*) payment
— **inicial** (*m.*) down payment
país (*m.*) country (nation)
— **de origen** (*m.*) country of origin
palabra (*f.*) word
paladar (*m.*) palate
pálido(a) pale
paliza (*f.*) spanking, beating
palpitación (*f.*) palpitation
pan (*m.*) bread
— **tostado** (*m.*) toast
pantalones (*m. pl.*) pants
pantimedias (*f. pl.*) pantyhose
pantorrilla (*f.*) calf
pañal (*m.*) diaper
— **desechable** (*m.*) disposable diaper
pañuelo de papel (*m.*) tissue
papa (*f.*) potato
papá (*m.*) father, dad

Papanicolau: examen de — (*m.*) Pap test (smear)
papas fritas (*f. pl.*) French fries
papel (*m.*) paper
paperas (*f. pl.*) mumps
papiloma (*m.*) papilloma
par (*m.*) pair, couple
para for, in order to, to
— **hoy mismo** for today
¿— **qué?** For what . . . ?, For what reason?, What for?, Why?
— **servirle.** (I'm) at your service.
— **ver si...** To see if . . .
parabrisas (*m. sing.*) windshield
parálisis (*f.*) paralysis
paralítico(a) paralyzed
paramédico(a) (*m., f.*) paramedic
pararse to stand up
parcial partial
parecer to seem, to look
pared (*f.*) wall
pareja (*f.*) pair, couple
parentesco (*m.*) relationship (*in a family*)
pariente (*m., f.*) relative
— **cercano(a)** (*m., f.*) close relative
parir to give birth
párpado (*m.*) eyelid
parroquial parochial
parte (*f.*) part
partera (*f.*) midwife
participar to take part, to participate
partida (*f.*) certificate
— **de bautismo** (*f.*) baptism certificate
— **de defunción** (*f.*) death certificate

— de ... dólares (*f.*) increment of . . . dollars
— de matrimonio (*f.*) marriage certificate
— de nacimiento (*f.*) birth certificate
parto (*m.*) delivery, childbirth
dolor de — (*m.*) labor pain
estar de — to be in labor
sala de — (*f.*) delivery room
pasado(a) last
pasado mañana the day after tomorrow
pasaporte (*m.*) passport
pasar to come in; to happen; to spend (*time*)
Pase. Come in.
pasársele a uno to pass; to forget, to slip one's mind
pasillo (*m.*) hallway
paso (*m.*) step
un — más a step further
pasta (*f.*) pasta
— de dientes (*f.*) toothpaste
— dentífrica (*f.*) toothpaste
pastel (*m.*) pie; cake
pastilla (*f.*) pill
— para el dolor (*f.*) painkiller
pasto (*m.*) marijuana (*coll.*)
pastor(a) (*m., f.*) pastor; person of the clergy
patada (*f.*) kick
patio (*m.*) backyard
patrón(ona) (*m., f.*) boss
patrono (*m.*) (*Cuba*) boss
PCP (*f.*) angel dust
pecho (*m.*) breast, chest
pediatra (*m., f.*) pediatrician
pediatría (*f.*) pediatrics
pedir (e:i) to ask for; to request

— **ayuda** to apply for aid
— **hora** to make an appointment
— **turno** to make an appointment
— **un favor** to ask a favor
Pida ver... Ask to see . . .

pegar to hit, to shoot, to strike
peligro (*m.*) danger
peligroso(a) dangerous
pelo (*m.*) hair
pelota (*f.*) ball
pelvis (*f.*) pelvis
pena (*f.*) penalty
penalidad (*f.*) penalty
pene (*m.*) penis
penicilina (*f.*) penicillin
pensar (e:ie) to think (about), to plan
— **(+ *inf.*)** to plan (to do something)
— **en eso** to think about that

pensión (*f.*) pension
— **alimenticia** (*f.*) child support, alimony

pensionado(a) retired
peor worse, worst
pequeño(a) small, little
pera (*f.*) pear
perder (e:ie) to lose
— **peso** to lose weight

pérdida (*f.*) loss
perdón pardon me, excuse me
perdonar to pardon, to forgive
perfecto(a) perfect
perfil (*m.*) side
perfume (*m.*) perfume
perico (*m.*) cocaine (*coll.*)
periódico (*m.*) newspaper

periodo (*m.*) menstruation, period
permanente permanent
permiso (*m.*) permission
— **de detención** (*m.*) warrant; order
— **de trabajo** (*m.*) work permit
permitido(a) allowable
pero but
peroné (*m.*) fibula
perro(a) (*m., f.*) dog
persona (*f.*) person
— **extraña** (*f.*) stranger
personal personal; (*m.*) staff, personnel
pertenencia (*f.*) belonging
pesado(a) heavy
pesar to weigh
pescado (*m.*) fish
pescuezo (*m.*) neck
peso (*m.*) weight
pestañas (*f. pl.*) eyelashes
pezón (*m.*) nipple
picado(a) decayed, carious
picadura (*f.*) cavity; bite
picante spicy
picazón (*f.*) itching
pico (*m.*) bit, small amount
pie (*m.*) foot
piedra (*f.*) stone; crack cocaine (*coll.*)
piel (*f.*) skin
pierna (*f.*) leg
pijama (*m.*) pajamas
píldora (*f.*) pill
pimiento (*m.*) pepper
piña (*f.*) pineapple
pinta (*f.*) pint

pintura (*f.*) paint
pinzas (*f. pl.*) tweezers
piorrea (*f.*) pyorrhea
piscina (*f.*) swimming pool
piso (*m.*) floor; story
pito (*m.*) marijuana (*coll.*)
placa (*f.*) plaque
placenta (*f.*) placenta
plancha (*f.*) iron
planificación (*f.*) planning
planilla (*f.*) form
planta del pie (*f.*) sole of the foot
plástico (*m.*) plastic
plazo (*m.*) term
pleuresía (*f.*) pleurisy
pobre poor
pobrecito(a) (*m., f.*) poor little thing (one)
poco(a) little, few
  — a poco little by little
  un — a little
pocos(as) few
poder (o:ue) to be able to, can
podiatra (*m., f.*) podiatrist
polen (*m.*) pollen
policía (*f.*) police (force); (*m., f.*) police officer, policeman; policewoman
policlínica (*f.*) clinic; hospital
polio, poliomielitis (*f.*) polio(myelitis)
póliza (*f.*) policy
pollo (*m.*) chicken
polvo (*m.*) cocaine (*coll.*)
  — de ángel (*m.*) angel dust
pomo (*m.*) bottle (*Cuba*)

poner to make, to put
— **una inyección** to give a shot
— **violento(a)** to make violent
ponerse to put on; to turn
— **azul** to turn blue
— **blanco(a)** to turn white
— **en contacto** to get in touch
— **pálido(a)** to turn pale
— **rojo(a)** to turn red
— **tenso(a)** to tense up
por through, for
— **ciento** percent
— **completo** completely
— **correo** by mail
¿— **cuánto tiempo...?** For how long . . .?
— **culpa de** because of
— **desgracia** unfortunately
— **día** daily; per day
— **ejemplo** for example
— **enfermedad** due to illness
— **eso** that's why, for that reason
— **favor** please
— **fin** finally
— **la boca** through the mouth
— **la mañana (tarde)** in the morning (afternoon)
— **la noche** at night
— **lo menos** at least
— **mí** for me, on my behalf
¿— **qué?** why?
— **semana** weekly; per week
— **suerte** luckily
— **supuesto** of course
— **un tiempo** for a while

— **unos segundos** for a few seconds
— **vía bucal** orally
— **vía oral** orally
porción (*f.*) portion, serving
poro (*m.*) pore
porque because
porro (*m.*) joint (*coll.*)
— **mortal** (*m.*) killer joint
portal (*m.*) porch
portarse to behave
— **mal** to misbehave
poseer to own
posibilidad (*f.*) possibility
posible possible
posiblemente possibly
posición (*f.*) position
postal postal
positivo(a) positive
posterior rear
postizo(a) false
postnatal postnatal
postre (*m.*) dessert
practicar to practice
precaución (*f.*) precaution
preferir (e:ie) to prefer
pregunta (*f.*) question
preguntar to ask (*a question*)
prematuro(a) premature
preñada pregnant (*coll.*)
prenatal prenatal
prendas (*f. pl.*) clothing
prender to react
preocupado(a) worried

preocupar(se) to worry
  — por to worry about
preparar to prepare
présbite farsighted
presentar to present, to file
  — una demanda to file a lawsuit
presente (*m.*) present
preservativo (*m.*) condom
presión (*f.*) blood pressure, presure
  — alta (*f.*) hypertension, high blood pressure
  — arterial (*f.*) blood pressure
preso(a) (*m., f.*) prisoner
préstamo (*m.*) loan
presupuesto (*m.*) budget
prevenir (e:ie) to prevent
prima (*f.*) premium
primario(a) primary
primavera (*f.*) spring
primero (*adv.*) first
  —(a) first (one)
primeros auxilios (*m. pl.*) first aid
primo(a) (*m., f.*) cousin
principal main
principio (*m.*) principle
privado(a) private
probable probable
probablemente probably
probar (o:ue) to try
probeta (*f.*) test tube
  bebé de — (*m.*) test-tube baby
problema (*m.*) problem
profesión (*f.*) profession
profundo(a) deep
programa (*m.*) program

prohibir to forbid, to prohibit
promedio (*m.*) average
pronto soon
  tan — como as soon as
propiedad (*f.*) property, asset
propio(a) itself, own
proporcionar to provide
próstata (*f.*) prostate gland
prostatitis (*f.*) prostatitis
proteger to protect
proteína (*f.*) protein
protestante Protestant
provenir (e:ie) to come from; to originate
provisional provisional
próximo(a) (*adj.*) next; (*m., f.*) next one
  la próxima vez next time
proyecto de la ciudad (*m.*) city (housing) project
prueba (*f.*) proof, test
psicólogo(a) (*m., f.*) psychologist
psiquiatra (*m., f.*) psychiatrist
psiquiátrico(a) psychiatric
publicar to publish
público(a) public
puede ser... it may be . . .
puente (*m.*) bridge
  — coronario (*m.*) (heart) bypass
puerta (*f.*) door
pues well
pujar to push (*during labor*)
pulgada (*f.*) inch
pullar to shoot up (*coll., Caribe*)
pulmón (*m.*) lung
pulmonía (*f.*) pneumonia

pulpa (*f.*) pulp
pulso (*m.*) pulse
puntada (*f.*) stitch
punto (*m.*) stitch, dot
punzada (*f.*) sharp pain
punzante sharp, stabbing
puñetazo (*m.*) punch
puño (*m.*) fist
pupila (*f.*) (eye) pupil
purgante (*m.*) purgative, cathartic
pus (*m.*) pus

Q

que that
  ¡— le vaya bien! Good luck!
  ¡— se mejore! Get well soon!
¡qué! how . . . !, what (a) . . . !
  ¡— bueno! That's great!
  ¡— suerte! How fortunate!, It's a good thing!, What luck!
¿qué? what?
  ¿— edad tiene(n)...? How old is/are . . . ?
  ¿— hora es? What time is it?
  ¿— más? What else?
  ¿— necesitas? What do you need?
  ¿— se le ofrece? What can I do for you?
  ¿— tal? How is it going?
  ¿— te pasa? What's the matter with you?
quebrarse (e:ie) to break, to fracture (*Méx.*)
quedar to be located
quedar(se) to remain, to stay
  — con to keep

— **paralítico(a)** to become paralyzed, to become crippled
— **quieto(a)** to sit (stay) still
— **sordo(a)** to go deaf
quehaceres del hogar (de la casa) (*m. pl.*) housework
queja (*f.*) complaint
quejarse to complain
quemadura (*f.*) burn
quemar(se) to burn (oneself)
querer (e:ie) to love, to want, to wish
— **decir** to mean
queso (*m.*) cheese
quiebra (*f.*) bankruptcy
¿quién? whom?, who?
quiste (*m.*) cyst
quieto(a) still
quijada (*f.*) jaw
quimioterapia (*f.*) chemotherapy
quiropráctico(a) (*m., f.*) chiropractor
quirúrgico(a) surgical
quitar(se) to take out, to remove
— **la ropa** to take off one's clothes
quizá(s) perhaps, maybe

R

rabadilla (*f.*) coccyx
rabí (*m.*) rabbi
rabino (*m.*) rabbi
radio (*m.*) radius
radiografía (*f.*) X-ray
radiología (*f.*) radiology
radiólogo(a) (*m., f.*) radiologist

raíz (*f.*) root
rápidamente rapidly
raquídea (*f.*) spinal anesthesia
raro(a) rare
rasguño (*m.*) scratch
rasurar(se) to shave
rato (*m.*) while
  — **libre** (*m.*) free time
ratón (*m.*) mouse
rayos equis (*m. pl.*) X-rays
raza (*f.*) race
reanimación (*f.*) revival
rebajar to lose weight
realizar to do, to carry out
recámara (*f.*) bedroom (*Méx.*)
recepcionista (*m., f.*) receptionist
recertificación (*f.*) recertification
receta (*f.*) prescription
recetado(a) prescribed
recetar to prescribe
recibir to receive
recibo (*m.*) receipt
recién new
  — **casado(a)** (*m., f.*) newlywed
  — **nacido(a)** (*m., f.*) newborn baby
recipiente (*m., f.*) recipient
reclusorio para menores (*m.*) juvenile hall
recomendar (e:ie) to recommend
reconciliación (*f.*) reconciliation
reconocer to examine; to recognize
recordar (o:ue) to remember
recto (*m.*) rectum
recuperación (*f.*) recovery
recuperarse to recover

recurrir (a) to turn (to)
reembolso (*m.*) refund
reevaluar to reevaluate
reformatorio (*m.*) reformatory
refresco (*m.*) soft drink, soda pop
refrigerador (*m.*) refrigerator
regalo (*m.*) gift, present
registración (*f.*) registration (*Méx.*)
registro (*m.*) registration
regla (*f.*) menstruation
reglamento (*m.*) rule
regresar to return, to come back
regularmente regularly
rehusar to refuse
relacionado(a) related
relaciones sexuales (*f. pl.*) sexual relations
  tener — to have sex
relajarse to relax (oneself)
reloj (*m.*) watch
remangarse to roll up one's sleeves
remedio (*m.*) medicine
renglón (*m.*) line (*on a paper or form*)
renta (*f.*) rent
renunciar to resign, to waive
reorientación vocacional (*f.*) vocational training
reparación (*f.*) repair
repollo (*m.*) cabbage
reproductivo(a) reproductive
requerido(a) required
resbalar to slip
resfriado(a) (*m.*) suffering from a cold
resfrío (*m.*) cold
residencia (*f.*) residence

residente (*m., f.*) resident
resollar to breath
resolver (o:ue) to solve
respiración (*f.*) breath
respirar to breathe
  Respire hondo. Take a deep breath., Breathe deeply.
respiratorio(a) respiratory
responsable responsible
respuesta (*f.*) answer
resto (*m.*) rest, remainder
resultado (*m.*) result
  dar — to work, to produce results
resumen (*m.*) summary
retención (*f.*) retention
retina (*f.*) retina
retirado(a) retired
retirarse to retire, to withdraw
retiro (*m.*) retirement
reumatismo (*m.*) rheumatism
reverso (*m.*) reverse, back (*of a page*)
revestir (e:i) to line
revisar to check
revisión (*f.*) review
revista (*f.*) magazine
riesgo (*m.*) risk
riñón (*m.*) kidney
ritmo (*m.*) rhythm
roca (*f.*) crack (*coll.*)
rodilla (*f.*) knee
rojo(a) red
romper to break
romper(se) to break, to fracture
  — la fuente to break water (*childbirth*)

ronchas (*f. pl.*) hives
ronco(a) hoarse
ronquera (*f.*) hoarseness
ropa (*f.*) clothes, clothing
— **interior** (*f.*) underwear
rótula (*f.*) patella
rubéola (*f.*) rubella
ruido (*m.*) noise, ringing (ear)

S

sábana (*f.*) sheet
saber to know (something)
sacar to pull out, to take out, to extract, to stick out
sacerdote (*m.*) priest
sal (*f.*) salt
sala (*f.*) living room, ward
— **de bebés** (*f.*) nursery
— **de cirugía** (*f.*) operating room
— **de emergencia** (*f.*) emergency room
— **de espera** (*f.*) waiting room
— **de estar** (*f.*) family room, den
— **de maternidad** (*f.*) maternity ward
— **de parto** (*f.*) delivery room
— **de rayos X** (*f.*) X-ray room
— **de recuperación** (*f.*) recovery room
— **de terapia física** (*f.*) physical theraphy room
— **de urgencia** (*f.*) emergency room
salario (*m.*) salary
saldo (*m.*) balance (*of a bank account*)
salir to leave, to go out
— **bien** to turn out okay

salirle un líquido a uno to have a discharge
saliva (*f.*) saliva
salpullido (*m.*) rash
salud (*f.*) health
saludo (*m.*) greeting
salvar to save
sangrar to bleed
sangre (*f.*) blood
sano(a) healthy
sarampión (*m.*) measles
sarna (*f.*) scabies
sarpullido (*m.*) rash
sarro (*m.*) tartar
sección (*f.*) section
  — **Protectora de Niños** (*f.*) Children's Protection Department
seco(a) dry
secreción (*f.*) secretion
secundario(a) secondary
  efecto secundario (*m.*) side effect
sed (*f.*) thirst
seda dental (*f.*) dental floss
sedante (*m.*) sedative, tranquilizer
sedativo (*m.*) tranquilizer
seguida: en — right away
seguir (e:i) to continue, to follow
según according to
segundo(a) second
  segundo nombre (*m.*) middle name
seguro (*m.*) insurance
  — **de hospitalización** (*m.*) hospital insurance
  — **de salud** (*m.*) health insurance
  — **de vida** (*m.*) life insurance

— **ferroviario** (*m.*) railroad insurance
— **médico** (*m.*) medical insurance
— **social** (*m.*) social security
seguro(a) sure, safe
semana (*f.*) week
la — próxima (entrante) next week
la — que viene next week
semanalmente weekly
semen (*m.*) semen
semestre (*m.*) semester
semiduro(a) medium hard
semiprivado(a) semiprivate
seno (*m.*) breast
sentado(a) sitting
sentar(se) (e:ie) to sit (down)
Siéntese. Sit down.
sentidos (*m. pl.*) senses
sentir (e:ie) que to regret that
Lo siento. I'm sorry.
sentir(se) (e:ie) to feel
señal (*f.*) sign; warning
señalar to indicate
señor (Sr.) (*m.*) Mr., sir, gentleman
señora (Sra.) (*f.*) Mrs., lady, Ma'am, Madam, wife
señorita (Srta.) (*f.*) Miss, young lady
separación (*f.*) separation
separado(a) separated
separar to separate
ser to be
— **cierto** to be true
— **querido** (*m.*) loved one
serio(a) serious

servicio (*m.*) bathroom; service
  — gratuito (*m.*) free service
servir (e:i) to serve
  para servirle at your service
sexo (*m.*) sex; gender
sexto(a) sixth
si if
  — es posible if possible
sí yes
sicosis (*f.*) psychosis
SIDA (Síndrome de Inmunodeficiencia Adquirida) (*m.*) AIDS
siempre always
sien (*f.*) temple
sífilis (*f.*) syphilis
sifilítico(a) (*adj.*) syphilitic
significar to mean
siguiente following, next
  lo — the following
silla (*f.*) chair
  — de ruedas (*f.*) wheelchair
sillita alta (*f.*) high chair
sillón (*m.*) armchair
similar similar
simple simple
simplemente simply
sin without
  — embargo however, nevertheless
  — falta without fail
  — hogar homeless
  — sal salt free
sinagoga (*f.*) synagogue, temple
síntoma (*m.*) symptom
siquiatría (*f.*) psychiatry

sirviente(a) (*m., f.*) servant
situación (*f.*) situation
sobre about, on
  — todo especially, above all
sobredosis (*f.*) overdose
sobrellevar to bear
sobrino(a) (*m., f.*) nephew; niece
social social
sofá (*m.*) sofa
sofocar(se) to suffocate (oneself)
sol (*m.*) sun; monetary unit of Peru
solamente only
solicitante (*m., f.*) applicant
solicitar to apply for
  Solicite ver... Ask to see . . .
solicitud (*f.*) application
solo(a) alone
sólo only
soltero(a) single
sombreado(a) shaded
Somos (+ *number*). There are (+ *number*) of us.
Son las (+ *time*). It's (+ *time*).
sonograma (*m.*) sonogram
sopa (*f.*) soup
soplo cardíaco (*m.*) (heart) murmur
sordera (*f.*) deafness
sordo(a) deaf; dull (*pain*)
sospecha (*f.*) suspicion
sospechar to suspect
sótano (*m.*) basement
su(s) your, his, her, their
subir to climb, to lift, to go up
  — de peso to gain weight
  subirse la manga(s) to roll up one's sleeve(s)

subsidio (*m.*) subsidy
subvención (*f.*) subsidy
suceder to happen
sudor (*m.*) sweat
suegro(a) (*m., f.*) father-in-law; mother-in-law
sueldo (*m.*) salary
suero (*m.*) I.V. (serum)
suerte (*f.*) luck
suficiente enough, sufficient
sufrir to suffer
— **del corazón** to have heart trouble
sugerencia (*f.*) suggestion
sugerir (e:ie) to suggest
suicidarse to commit suicide
sulfa (*f.*) sulfa
supervisor(a) (*m., f.*) supervisor
superviviente (*m., f.*) survivor
suplementario(a) supplemental
supositorio (*m.*) suppository
supuración (*f.*) pus
suscripción (*f.*) subscription
susto (*m.*) fright
suyo(a) your (*form.*), his, her, their

T

tabaco (*m.*) tobacco
tableta (*f.*) tablet
tal vez perhaps
talco para bebé (*m.*) baby powder
talón (*m.*) heel
talonario de cheques (*m.*) checkbook
tamaño (*m.*) size
también also

tampoco either, neither
tan as
 —... como as . . . as
 — pronto como as soon as
tanto tiempo so long
tantos(as) so many, so much
tapa de seguridad (*f.*) safety cap, safety cover
tapado(a) constipated
tapar to cover, to block
taquicardia (*f.*) tachycardia
tarde (*f.*) afternoon; (*adv.*) late
 más — later
tareas de la casa (*f. pl.*) housework
tarjeta (*f.*) card
 — de crédito (*f.*) credit card
 — de inmigración (*f.*) immigration card
 — de seguro médico (*f.*) medical insurance card
 — de Seguro Social (*f.*) Social Security card
tarso (*m.*) tarsus
taza (*f.*) cup
techo (*m.*) ceiling
técnico(a) (*m., f.*) technician
tejido (*m.*) tissue
 — graso (*m.*) fatty tissue
tela (*f.*) cloth
teléfono (*m.*) telephone
televisor (*m.*) television (set), TV
temblor (*m.*) tremor, shaking
temer to be afraid, to fear
temperatura (*f.*) temperature
 la — pasa de... the temperature is over . . .
temporal temporary
temprano early

tendencia (*f.*) tendency
tener to have
— **a mano** to keep at hand
—**... años** to be . . . years old
— **casa propia** to own a house
— **cuidado** to be careful
— **derecho a (+ *inf.*)** to have the right to (do something)
— **dolor** to be in pain
— **dolor de espalda** to have a backache
— **en cuenta** to keep in mind
— **hambre** to be hungry
— **mal olor (peste)** to have a bad odor
— **miedo** to be afraid
(no) — importancia to (not) matter
— **prisa** to be in a hurry
— **que (+ *inf.*)** to have to (do something)
— **razón** to be right
— **sueño** to be sleepy
— **suerte** to be lucky
— **un flujo** to have a discharge
tensión (*f.*) blood pressure; tension
— **familiar** (*f.*) family tension
terapia (*f.*) therapy
— **física** (*f.*) physical therapy
tercero(a) third
terminar to finish, to be done
término (*m.*) term
termómetro (*m.*) thermometer
terremoto (*m.*) earthquake
terrible terrible
testículo (*m.*) testicle
testigo (*m.*, *f.*) witness
tétano(s) (*m.*) tetanus

tete (*m.*) pacifier (*Cuba*)
tía (*f.*) aunt
tibia (*f.*) tibia
tibio(a) lukewarm, tepid
tiempo (*m.*) time
— **libre** (*m.*) free time
tienda (*f.*) store; shop
tijeras (*f. pl.*) scissors
tímpano (*m.*) eardrum
tina (*f.*) bathtub (*Méx.*)
tinta (*f.*) ink
tinte (*m.*) dye
tintura de yodo (*f.*) iodine
tío (*m.*) uncle
tipo (*m.*) type
tiroides (*m. sing.*) thyroid
glándula — (*f. sing.*) thyroid gland
título (*m.*) title
toallita (*f.*) washcloth
tobilleras (*f.*) socks (*Méx.*)
tobillo (*m.*) ankle
tocar to touch
tocar a la puerta to knock at the door
todavía still, yet
todo all, everything
— **el día** all day long
— **eso** all that
— **lo posible** everything possible
— **los días** every day
todo(a) all
tomacorrientes (*m. sing.*) electrical outlet, socket
tomar to drink, to take
— **asiento** to have a seat

— **la presión** to take the blood pressure
— **la tensión** to take the blood pressure
— **una decisión** to make a decision
— **un idioma** to take (study) a language
Tome asiento. Have a seat.
tomate (*m.*) tomato
tórax (*m.*) thorax
torcer(se) (o:ue) to twist
torcido(a) crooked
torniquete (*m.*) tourniquet
toronja (*f.*) grapefruit
tortilla (*f.*) tortilla
tos (*f.*) cough
— **convulsiva** (*f.*) whooping cough
— **ferina** (*f.*) whooping cough, pertussis
toser to cough
tostada (*f.*) toast
total (*m.*) total
trabajador(a) (*m., f.*) worker
— **agrícola** (*m., f.*) farm worker
— **social** (*m., f.*) social worker
trabajar to work
— **medio día** to work part-time
— **parte del tiempo** to work part-time
— **por cuenta propia** to be self-employed
— **por su cuenta** to be self-employed
— **tiempo completo** to work full-time
trabajo (*m.*) work, job
— **de la casa** (*m.*) housework
traductor(a) (*m., f.*) translator
traer to bring
tragar to swallow
trámites de divorcio (*m. pl.*) divorce proceedings

tranquilizante (*m.*) tranquilizer
transfusión (*f.*) transfusion
transmitido(a) transmitted
  — a través del contacto sexual sexually transmitted
trasplante de corazón (*m.*) heart transplant
trastorno nervioso (*m.*) nervous disorder
tratamiento (*m.*) treatment
tratar (de) to treat, to deal with; to try
travesura (*f.*) mischief, prank
travieso(a) mischievous, restless
tribunal (*m.*) court
trimestre (*m.*) quarter (three months)
tripas (*f. pl.*) belly; intestines
tripear to take drugs (*coll.*)
trompa (*f.*) tube
trompada (*f.*) punch
tuberculina (*f.*) tuberculin
tuberculosis (*f.*) tuberculosis
tubo (*m.*) tube
tuerto(a) one-eyed
tumor (*m.*) tumor
tupido(a) constipated
turno (*m.*) appointment
tutor(a) (*m., f.*) guardian

U

úlcera (*f.*) ulcer
últimamente lately
último(a) last
  la última vez the last time
ultrasonido (*m.*) ultrasound
ultrasonografía (*f.*) ultrasound

ungüento (*m.*) ointment
único(a) only
unidad (*f.*) unit
— **de cuidados intensivos** (*f.*) intensive care unit
un, una a, an
unos about, some
urea alta (*f.*) uremia
uremia (*f.*) uremia
uretra (*f.*) urethra
urgente urgent
urgentemente urgently
úrico(a) uric
urología (*f.*) urology
urólogo(a) (*m., f.*) urologist
urticaria (*f.*) hives
usado(a) used
usar to wear, to use
uso (*m.*) use
útero (*m.*) uterus
útil useful
utilizar to use
uva (*f.*) grape
úvula (*f.*) uvula

V

va a haber... there is going to be . . .
vacío(a) empty
vacunado(a) vaccinated
vacunar to vaccinate, to immunize
vagina (*f.*) vagina
vaginal vaginal
vaginitis (*f.*) vaginitis

valer to be worth
valor (*m.*) value
Vamos a ver. Let's see.
varicela (*f.*) chickenpox
várices (*f. pl.*) varicose veins
variedad (*f.*) variety
varios(as) several
varón (*m.*) male, boy
vasectomía (*f.*) vasectomy
vaselina (*f.*) Vaseline
vasito (*m.*) little glass, cup
vaso (*m.*) glass
veces (*f. pl.*) times
  a — sometimes
  algunas — sometimes
  muchas — many times
vecino(a) (*m., f.*) neighbor
vegetal (*m.*) vegetable
veinte twenty
vejiga (*f.*) bladder
vena (*f.*) vein
  — varicosa (*f.*) varicose vein
vencer to expire
venda (*f.*) bandage
vendaje (*m.*) bandage
vendar to bandage
vender to sell
veneno (*m.*) poison
venéreo(a) venereal
venir (e:ie) to come
ventaja (*f.*) advantage
ventana (*f.*) window
  — de la nariz (*f.*) nostril
  — nasal (*f.*) nostril

ver to see
  vamos a — let's see
verano (*m.*) summer
verbo (*m.*) verb
verdad true
  ¿verdad? right?
verdadero(a) true, real
verde green
verdoso(a) greenish
verificación (*f.*) verification
verificar to verify
verruga (*f.*) wart
verse to look, to seem
vértebra (*f.*) vertebra
vesícula (*f.*) vesicle
  — biliar (*f.*) gallbladder
  — seminal (*f.*) seminal vesicle
vestido (*m.*) dress
vez (*f.*) time
  de — en cuando from time to time
  una — once
víctima (*f.*) victim
vida (*f.*) life
viejo(a) (*m., f.*) elderly man, elderly woman; (*adj.*) old
vientre (*m.*) abdomen
VIH (virus de inmunodeficiencia humana) (*m.*) HIV (human immunodeficiency virus)
vino (*m.*) wine
violencia doméstica (*f.*) domestic violence
violento(a) violent, strenuous
viruela (*f.*) smallpox
virus (*m.*) virus

— de inmunodeficiencia humana (*m.*) human immunodeficiency virus
visa de estudiante (*f.*) student visa
visitador(a) social (*m., f.*) social worker who makes home visits
visitar to visit
vista (*f.*) court hearing; vision; view
corto(a) de — nearsighted
vitamina (*f.*) vitamin
viudo(a) (*m., f.*) widow, widowed, widower
vivienda (*f.*) home, lodging
vivir to live
vocabulario (*m.*) vocabulary
voltearse to turn over (*Méx.*)
volver (o:ue) to come (go) back, to return
volverse (o:ue) to turn over
vomitar to throw up

Y

y and
ya already, now
— está. That's it.
— lo sé. I know (it).
— no no longer
¿— terminamos? Are we finished already?
yerba (*f.*) marijuana (*coll.*)
yerno (*m.*) son-in-law
yeso (*m.*) cast
yo mismo(a) myself
yodo (*m.*) iodine
yogur (*m.*) yogurt

Z

zapatilla (*f.*) slipper
zapato (*m.*) shoe
zona postal (*f.*) zip code, postal code

English–Spanish

A

a un, una
— **day** al día
— **week** a la semana
— **while later** al rato
able capacitado(a)
abdomen vientre (*m.*), barriga (*f.*), abdomen (*m.*)
abortion aborto (*m.*)
about (*prep.*) acerca de, sobre; (*approximately*) hace como..., unos(as)
above sobre
— **all** sobre todo
abscess absceso (*m.*)
absent ausente
abstinence abstinencia (*f.*)
abuse maltrato (*m.*); maltratar
accept aceptar
accessory accesorio (*m.*)
accident accidente (*m.*)
according to de acuerdo con, según
accusation denuncia (*f.*)
accuse denunciar, acusar
ache dolor (*m.*); doler (o:ue)
acid ácido (*m.*)
acidity acidez (*f.*)
acne acné (*m.*)
acquainted: to be — with conocer
add añadir
addicted adicto(a)
address dirección (*f.*), domicilio (*m.*)

adhesive tape cinta adhesiva (*f.*), esparadrapo (*m.*)
adjective adjetivo (*m.*)
administrator administrador(a) (*m., f.*)
admission admisión (*f.*)
admit (to a hospital) ingresar, internar
adult adulto(a) (*m., f.*)
advance adelanto (*m.*)
advantage ventaja (*f.*)
 take — of aprovechar
advice consejo (*m.*)
advise avisar, hacer saber, aconsejar
affair cosa (*f.*)
affect afectar
affirmative afirmativo(a)
after después (de)
afternoon tarde (*f.*)
afterward después (de)
again otra vez, de nuevo
against contra
age edad (*f.*)
agency agencia (*f.*)
ago: a month — hace un mes
 How long — . . . ? ¿Cuánto tiempo hace...?
agree estar de acuerdo
agreeable ameno(a)
agreement acuerdo (*m.*)
aha ajá
aid ayuda (*f.*)
 — to Families with Dependent Children (AFDC) ayuda a familias con niños (*f.*)
AIDS SIDA (Síndrome de Inmunodeficiencia Adquirida) (*m.*)
air aire (*m.*)

air conditioning aire acondicionado (*m.*)
alcohol alcohol (*m.*)
alcoholic alcohólico(a)
Alcoholics Anonymous Alcohólicos Anónimos
alimony pensión alimenticia (*f.*)
all todo(a), todos(as)
 — day long todo el día
 — that todo eso
allergic alérgico(a)
allergy alergia (*f.*)
allow dejar
allowable permitido(a)
almost casi
alone solo(a)
already ya
also también, asimismo
always siempre
ambulance ambulancia (*f.*)
American (North American) americano(a), norteamericano(a)
among entre
amount cantidad (*f.*)
 small — pico (*m.*)
amphetamine anfetamina (*f.*)
amputate amputar
an un, una
anabolic steroids esteroides anabólicos (*m. pl.*)
analgesics analgésicos (*m. pl.*)
analysis análisis (*m.*)
and y
anemia anemia (*f.*)
anemic anémico(a)
anesthesia anestesia (*f.*)
anesthesiologist anestesiólogo(a) (*m., f.*)

anesthesiology anestesiología (*f.*)
aneurysm aneurisma (m.)
angel dust PCP (*f.*), polvo de ángel (*m.*)
angina angina (*f.*)
angioplasty angioplastia, angioplastía (*f.*)
angry enojado(a)
ankle tobillo (*m.*)
annoyed molesto(a)
annuity anualidad (*f.*)
another otro(a)
answer contestar; contestación (*f.*), respuesta (*f.*)
antacid antiácido (*m.*)
antibacterial antibacteriano(a)
antibiotic antibiótico (*m.*)
anticoagulant anticoagulante (*m.*)
antidepressant antidepresivo (*m.*)
antidrug antidroga
antihistamine antihistamínico (*m.*)
anus ano (*m.*)
anxiety ansiedad (*f.*), angustia (*f.*)
any algún(una), cualquier(a)
anybody, anyone alguien, nadie
anything algo
  — else? ¿Algo más?
anyway de todos modos
apartment apartamento (*m.*)
apparatus aparato (*m.*)
appear aparecer
appendicitis apendicitis (*f.*)
appetite apetito (*m.*)
apple manzana (*f.*)
applicant solicitante (*m., f.*)
application solicitud (*f.*)

apply (for) solicitar, aplicar
— **for aid** pedir (e:i) ayuda
appointment cita (*f.*), turno (*m.*)
approach acercarse
approval aprobación (*f.*)
arm brazo (*m.*)
armchair sillón (*m.*)
around alrededor (de)
arrangement arreglo (*m.*)
arrest arrestar, detener
arrive llegar
artery arteria (*f.*)
arthritis artritis (*f.*)
article artículo (*m.*)
artificial artificial
as como
— **. . . as** tan... como
— **of** a partir de
— **soon as** en cuanto, tan pronto como
— **soon as possible** lo más pronto posible, cuanto antes
ask preguntar
— **a favor** pedir (e:i) un favor
— **a question** preguntar
— **for** pedir (e:i)
— **questions** hacer preguntas
— **to see . . .** Solicite ver... , pida ver
asleep dormido(a)
aspirin aspirina (*f.*)
asset propiedad (*f.*)
assistant asistente (*m., f.*)
asthma asma (*f.* but **el asma**)
asthmatic asmático(a)
astigmatism astigmatismo (*m.*)

at en, a
— **(+ *time*)** a la(s) (+ *time*)
— **first** al principio
— **home** en casa
— **least** por lo menos
— **midday** a (al) mediodía
— **midnight** a (la) medianoche
— **night** por la noche
— **present** ahora
— **the beginning** al principio de
— **the bottom of the page** al pie de la página
— **the end of** al final de
— **the moment** en este momento
— **the present time** actualmente
— **your service** para servirle
atmosphere ambiente (*m.*)
attack ataque (*m.*)
attend asistir
aunt tía (*f.*)
authority autoridad (*f.*)
authorization autorización (*f.*)
authorize autorizar
autumn otoño (*m.*)
available disponible
avenue avenida (*f.*)
average promedio (*m.*)
avoid evitar
awake despierto(a)

B

baby bebé (*m.*), bebito (*m.*)

— **bottle** biberón (*m.*), mamadera (*f.*), mamila (*f.*) (*Méx.*)
— **carriage** cochecito (*m.*)
— **food** comidita de bebé (*f.*)
— **lotion** loción para bebé (*f.*)
— **powder** talco para bebé (*m.*)

back espalda (*f.*); (*of a page*) reverso (*m.*); (*adj.*) atrasado(a)
on the — al dorso

backbone columna vertebral (*f.*)

backward hacia atrás

backyard patio (*m.*)

bad malo(a)

badly mal

bail fianza (*f.*)

balance saldo (*m.*)

balanced balanceado(a)

ball pelota (*f.*)

balloon (*drug dosage*) globo (*m.*)

bandage venda (*f.*), vendaje (*m.*)

band-aid curita (*f.*)

bank banco (*m.*)

bankruptcy bancarrota (*f.*)

baptism certificate certificado de bautismo (*m.*), fe de bautismo (*f.*), inscripción de bautismo (*f.*), partida de bautismo (*f.*)

barbiturate barbitúrico (*m.*)

barely apenas

basement sótano (*m.*)

basic básico(a)

bathe bañar

bathroom baño (*m.*), escusado (*m.*), excusado (*m.*) (*Méx.*), servicio (*m.*), cuarto de baño (*m.*)

bathtub bañadera (*f.*), bañera (*f.*) (*Puerto Rico*), tina (*f.*) (*Méx.*)
battery batería (*f.*)
be ser, estar
— **able** poder (o:ue)
— **acquainted with (*a person, a place*)** conocer
— **admitted** ingresar
— **afraid** temer, tener miedo
— **born** nacer
— **called** llamarse
— **careful** tener cuidado
— **done** terminar
— **embarrassed** darle vergüenza a uno
— **enough** alcanzar
— **free on bail** estar en libertad bajo fianza
— **free on probation** estar en libertad condicional
— **frightened** asustarse
— **glad** alegrarse (de)
— **going to (do something)** ir a (+ *inf.*)
— **hungry** tener hambre
— **in a hurry** tener prisa
— **in charge (of)** encargarse (de)
— **in jail** estar preso(a)
— **in pain** tener dolor
— **lacking something** faltarle algo a uno
— **located** quedar
— **lucky** tener suerte
— **named** llamarse
— **nobody's business** no importarle a nadie
— **pleasing to** gustar
— **raised** criarse
— **right** tener razón

— **scared** asustarse
— **sleepy** tener sueño
— **tight** apretar (e:ie)
— **true** ser cierto
— **unemployed (out of work)** estar sin trabajo
— **worth** valer
— **wrong** estar equivocado(a)
— **. . . years old** tener ... años
beans frijoles (*m. pl.*), habichuelas (*f. pl.*) (*Puerto Rico*)
bear aguantar, sobrellevar
beat (*heart*) latir
beating paliza (*f.*)
because porque
— **of** por culpa de
become convertirse, ponerse
— **paralyzed (crippled)** quedarse paralítico(a)
bed cama (*f.*)
bedpan chata (*f.*), cuña (*f.*)
bedroom cuarto (*m.*), dormitorio (*m.*), habitación (*f.*), recámara (*f.*) (*Méx.*)
bedtime: at — al acostarse
beer cerveza (*f.*)
before (*adv.*) antes; (*prep.*) antes (de)
— **sleeping** antes de dormir
begin comenzar (e:ie), empezar (e:ie)
behave comportarse
believe creer
belonging pertenencia (*f.*)
belt cinto (*m.*), cinturón (*m.*)
bend doblar
benefit beneficio (*m.*)

benign benigno(a)
besides además (de)
best mejor, lo mejor
the — thing lo mejor
better mejor
between entre
beverage bebida (*f.*)
alcoholic — bebida alcohólica (*f.*)
bib babero (*m.*)
big grande
bilingual bilingüe
bill cuenta (*f.*)
biopsy biopsia (*f.*)
birth natalidad (*f.*), nacimiento (*m.*)
— certificate certificado de nacimiento (*m.*), inscripción de nacimiento (*f.*) (*Cuba*), partida de nacimiento (*f.*)
— control anticonceptivo(a) (*adj.*)
— mark mancha en la piel (*f.*)
to give — dar a luz, parir
bit pico (*m.*)
bite morder (o:ue); picadura (*f.*)
black negro(a)
blackhead espinilla (*f.*)
bladder vejiga (*f.*)
— stones cálculos en la vejiga (*m. pl.*)
bland blando(a)
blank space espacio en blanco (*m.*)
blanket frazada (*f.*), cobija (*f.*), manta (*f.*)
bleach lejía (*f.*)
bleed sangrar
bleeding pérdida de sangre (*f.*)
blind ciego(a)
blindness ceguera (*f.*)

blister ampolla (*f.*)
bloated aventado(a), lleno(a) de gases
block cuadra (*f.*); tapar
blood sangre (*f.*)
— **bank** banco de sangre (*m.*)
— **count** conteo (*m.*)
— **pressure** presión (*f.*), presión arterial (*f.*), tensión (*f.*)
— **relative** pariente cercano(a) (*m., f.*)
— **test** análisis de sangre (*m.*)
blouse blusa (*f.*)
blue azul
blurry borroso(a)
body cuerpo (*m.*)
boiling hirviendo
bond bono (*m.*)
bone hueso (*m.*)
bonnet gorro (*m.*)
bookcase estante (*m.*)
boss jefe (*m., f.*), patrón(ona) (*m., f.*), patrono (*m.*) (*Cuba*)
both los (las) dos
bothered molesto(a)
bottle frasco (*m.*), botella (*f.*), pomo (*m.*) (*Cuba*)
bowel movement: to have a — mover el vientre, obrar, defecar, evacuar (*Méx.*), hacer caca (*coll.*)
box caja (*f.*), cuadro (*m.*), cuadrado (*m.*)
boy niño (*m.*), varón (*m.*), muchacho (*m.*)
boyfriend novio (*m.*)
braces (dental) frenos (*m. pl.*)
brain cerebro (*m.*)
bread pan (*m.*)

break descomponerse, fracturar(se), quebrarse (e:ie) (*Méx.*), romperse
— **water (childbirth)** romperse la fuente
breakfast desayuno (*m.*)
breast seno (*m.*), pecho (*m.*)
breath aliento (m.), respiración (*f.*)
breathe respirar, resollar
bridge puente (*m.*)
brief breve
bring traer
broccoli bróculi (*m.*)
brochure folleto (*m.*)
broken down descompuesto(a)
broker's fee honorario de corredor (*m.*)
bronchitis bronquitis (*f.*)
bronchoscopy broncoscopia, broncoscopía (*f.*)
brother hermano (*m.*)
brother-in-law cuñado (*m.*)
bruise moretón (*m.*), morado (*m.*), cardenal (*m.*) (*Cuba*)
brush cepillo (*m.*); cepillar(se)
— **one's teeth** cepillarse los dientes
buddy compañero(a) (*m., f.*)
budget presupuesto (*m.*)
bump (on the head) chichón (*m.*)
bunion juanete (*m.*)
burden carga (*f.*)
burglar ladrón(ona) (*m., f.*)
burn arder, quemar(se); quemadura (*f.*)
burning ardor (*m.*)
burp eructar
business office oficina de pagos (*f.*)
busy ocupado(a)
but pero

butter mantequilla (*f.*)
buttock(s) nalga(s) (*f.*), asentadera(s) (*f.*)
button botón (*m.*)
buy comprar
by por
 — **mail** por correo
 — **the hand** de la mano
bye chau
bypass: heart — puente coronario (*m.*)

C

cabbage col (*f.*), repollo (*m.*)
caffeine cafeína (*f.*)
cake pastel (*m.*)
calcaneus calcáneo (*m.*)
calcium calcio (*m.*)
calf pantorrilla (*f.*)
call llamar
called llamado(a)
calm calma (*f.*); calmar
 — **down** calmar(se)
calorie caloría (*f.*)
can (be able to) poder (o:ue)
cancer cáncer (*m.*)
candy dulce (*m.*), caramelo (*m.*)
cane bastón (*m.*)
canine canino (*m.*)
cap gorro (*m.*)
capsule cápsula (*f.*)
car auto(móvil) (*m.*), carro (*m.*), coche (*m.*), máquina (*f.*) (*Cuba*)
carbohydrate carbohidrato (*m.*)
card tarjeta (*f.*)

cardiogram cardiograma (*m.*)
cardiologist cardiólogo(a) (*m., f.*)
cardiology cardiología (*f.*)
care cuidado (*m.*)
careful: to be — tener cuidado
carious picado(a), cariado(a)
carpus carpo (*m.*)
carry llevar
  — out llevar a cabo
case caso (*m.*)
  — history información sobre el caso (*f.*)
  in — of en caso de
  in that — en ese caso
cash efectivo (*m.*)
  — a check cambiar (cobrar) un cheque
  in — al contado, en efectivo
cashier cajero(a) (*m., f.*)
cast yeso (*m.*), escayola (*f.*) (*España*)
CAT scan escanograma (*m.*)
cataracts cataratas (*f. pl.*)
cathartic purgante (*m.*)
Catholic católico(a)
cause causa (*f.*); causar
cavity picadura (*f.*), caries (*f.*)
ceiling techo (*m.*)
cement cemento (*m.*)
cent centavo (*m.*), chavo (*m.*) (*Puerto Rico*)
center centro (*m.*)
cereal cereal (*m.*)
cerebrum cerebro (*m.*)
certain cierto(a), seguro(a)
certainly ciertamente
certificate certificado (*m.*), partida (*f.*)

— **of deposit (CD)** certificado de depósito (*m.*)
cervix cérvix (*f.*)
cesarean cesáreo(a)
chair silla (*f.*)
chancre chancro (*m.*)
change cambiar(se); cambio (*m.*)
— **into** convertirse (e:ie) en
— **jobs** cambiar de trabajo
chapter capítulo (*m.*)
charge cobrar
cheap barato(a)
check examinar, chequear, revisar; cheque (*m.*)
— **off** marcar
checkbook talonario de cheques (*m.*), chequera (*f.*) (*Cuba y Puerto Rico*)
checking account cuenta de cheques (*f.*), cuenta corriente (*f.*)
checkup chequeo (*m.*), examen (*m.*)
give a — hacer un examen
cheek cachete (*m.*), mejilla (*f.*)
cheese queso (*m.*)
chemotherapy quimioterapia (*f.*)
chest pecho (*m.*)
chest of drawers cómoda (*f.*)
chew masticar, mascar
chicken pollo (*m.*)
chickenpox varicela (*f.*)
child niño(a) (*m., f.*)
— **care license** licencia para cuidar niños (*f.*)
— **support** pensión alimenticia (*f.*)
childbirth parto (*m.*)
children hijos (*m.*), chicos(as) (*m., f.*), niños(as) (*m., f.*)

—'s **Protection Department** Sección Protectora de Niños (*f.*), Departamento de Protección de Niños (*m.*)
chills escalofríos (*m. pl.*)
chin barbilla (*f.*)
chiropractor quiropráctico(a) (*m., f.*)
chlamydia clamidia (*f.*)
chocolate chocolate (*m.*)
choke atragantarse
cholesterol colesterol (*m.*)
choose escoger, elegir (e:i)
Christmas Navidad (*f.*)
church iglesia (*f.*)
cigarette cigarrillo (*m.*)
circulation circulación (*f.*)
citizen ciudadano(a) (*m., f.*)
citizenship ciudadanía (*f.*)
city ciudad (*f.*)
— **(housing) project** proyecto de la ciudad (*m.*)
class clase (*f.*), curso (*m.*)
clavicle clavícula (*f.*)
clean limpiar; limpio(a)
cleaning limpieza (*f.*)
clearly claramente
clergy (person) pastor(a) (*m., f.*)
clerk empleado(a) (*m., f.*)
client cliente(a) (*m., f.*)
climb subir
clinic clínica (*f.*)
clogged obstruido(a)
close cerrar (e:ie); (*nearby*) cerca
closed cerrado(a)
clot embolia (*f.*), coágulo (*m.*)

clothes ropa (*f.*)
clothing ropa (*f.*), prendas (*f. pl.*)
coagulation coágulo (*m.*)
coagulum coágulo (*m.*)
coat abrigo (*m.*)
cocaine cocaína (*f.*), coca (*f.*), perico (*m.*) (*coll.*), polvo (*m.*) (*coll.*)
coccyx rabadilla (*f.*), cóccix (*m.*)
cockroach cucaracha (*f.*)
codeine codeína (*f.*)
coffee café (*m.*)
cognate cognado (*m.*)
coin moneda (*f.*)
cold catarro (*m.*), resfrío (*m.*), resfriado (*m.*); (*adj.*) frío(a)
  to have a — estar resfriado(a), estar acatarrado(a)
colic cólico (*m.*)
colitis colitis (*f.*), inflamación del intestino grueso (*f.*)
collide chocar
colon colon (*m.*)
colonoscopy colonoscopia, colonoscopía (*f.*)
color blindness daltonismo (*m.*)
coloscopy colonoscopia, colonoscopía (*f.*)
come venir, provenir
  — back regresar
  — from provenir
  — in pasar, entrar
comfortable cómodo(a)
commercial comercial
commission comisión (*f.*)
commit cometer
  — suicide suicidarse

common común
common-law marriage concubinato (*m.*)
commute ir y venir
companion compañero(a) (*m., f.*)
company compañía (*f.*)
compassion compasión (*f.*)
compare comparar
complain quejarse
complaint queja (*f.*)
complete completo(a); completar
completely completamente, por completo
complication complicación (*f.*)
compress compresa (*f.*)
conceive concebir (e:i)
condom condón (*m.*), preservativo (*m.*)
confidential confidencial
confirm confirmar
conjunctivitis conjuntivitis (*f.*)
consecutive consecutivo(a)
consent consentimiento (*m.*)
consist (of) consistir (en)
constantly constantemente
constipated estreñido(a), tapado(a), tupido(a)
consult consultar
consume consumir
contact contacto (*m.*)
— **lenses** lentes de contacto (*m. pl.*)
contagious contagioso(a)
contain contener
continue seguir (e:i), continuar
contraceptive (*adj.*) anticonceptivo(a); anticonceptivo (*m.*)
contraction contracción (*f.*)
control control (*m.*); controlar

convalescent convaleciente
convenience comodidad (*f.*), conveniencia (*f.*)
conversation conversación (*f.*)
convince convencer
convulsions convulsiones (*f. pl.*)
cook cocinar; cocinero(a) (*m., f.*)
— **(prepare) dinner** hacer la comida
cookie galletita (*f.*), galletica (*f.*) (*Cuba*)
cooperate cooperar
coordinator coordinador(a) (*m., f.*)
copy copia (*f.*)
correct correcto(a)
correctly correctamente
cosmetics cosméticos (*m. pl.*)
cost costar (o:ue); costo (*m.*)
cough tos (*f.*); toser
— **syrup** jarabe para la tos (*m.*)
count contar (o:ue); conteo (*m.*)
country campo (m.); (*nation*) país (*m.*)
— **of origin** país de origen (*m.*)
county condado (*m.*)
couple par (*m.*), pareja (*f.*)
course curso (*m.*)
of — cómo no, por supuesto
court hearing vista (*f.*)
courthouse juzgado (*m.*), tribunal (*m.*)
cousin primo(a) (*m., f.*)
cover cubrir, tapar
covered cubierto(a)
crack crac (*m.*), piedra (*f.*) (*coll.*), roca (*f.*) (*coll.*), coca cocinada (*f.*) (*coll.*)
cradle cuna (*f.*)
cramp calambre (*m.*)
crawl gatear, andar a gatas

cream crema (*f.*)
credit card tarjeta de crédito (*f.*)
crib cuna (*f.*)
crime crimen (*m.*), delito (*m.*)
crippled inválido(a)
crisis crisis (*f.*)
crooked torcido(a)
cross cruz (*f.*)
cross-eyed bizco(a)
croup crup (*m.*), garrotillo (*m.*)
crown corona (*f.*)
crutch muleta (*f.*)
cry llorar
cultural cultural
cup taza (*f.*), vasito (*m.*)
cure curar; cura (*f.*)
cured curado(a)
currently actualmente
curtain cortina (*f.*)
custody custodia (*f.*)
cut cortadura (*f.*), cortada (*f.*) (*Méx., Cuba*)
— **(oneself)** cortar(se)
— **down** disminuir
cyst quiste (*m.*)

D

dad padre (*m.*), papá (*m.*)
daily (*adv.*) al día, diariamente; (*adj.*) diario(a), por día
damage daño (*m.*); dañar
danger peligro (*m.*)
dangerous peligroso(a)
dark oscuridad (*f.*)

data datos (*m. pl.*)
date fecha (*f.*)
— **of birth** fecha de nacimiento (*f.*)
daughter hija (*f.*)
— **-in-law** nuera (*f.*)
day día (*m.*)
— **after tomorrow** pasado mañana
— **before yesterday** anteayer
on the following — al día siguiente
deaf sordo(a)
go — quedarse sordo(a)
deafness sordera (*f.*)
death muerte (*f.*)
— **certificate** certificado de defunción (*m.*), inscripción de defunción (*f.*), partida de defunción (*f.*)
debt deuda (*f.*)
decayed picado(a), cariado(a)
deceased fallecido(a)
decide decidir
decision decisión (*f.*)
decongestants descongestionantes (*m. pl.*)
deduct descontar (o:ue)
deductible deducible
deduction deducción (*f.*)
deep (*adv.*) hondo, (*adj.*) hondo(a), profundo(a)
deform deformar
degree grado (*m.*)
deliver entregar
delivery (*birth*) parto (*m.*), alumbramiento (*m.*)
— **room** sala de parto (*f.*)
den sala de estar (*f.*)
denied denegado(a)

dental dental
  — **floss** hilo dental (*m.*), seda dental (*f.*)
  — **surgeon** odontólogo(a) (*m., f.*)
dentine dentina (*f.*)
dentist dentista (*m., f.*), odontólogo(a) (*m., f.*)
denture dentadura postiza (*f.*)
department departamento (*m.*)
depend depender
dependent dependiente (*m., f.*)
depression depresión (*f.*)
dermatologist dermatólogo(a) (*m., f.*)
desk escritorio (*m.*)
dessert postre (*m.*)
destroy destruir
detachment desprendimiento (*m.*)
detergent detergente (*m.*)
determine determinar
detoxification desintoxicación (*f.*)
develop desarrollar
diabetes diabetes (*f.*)
diabetic diabético(a)
diagnose diagnosticar
diagnosis diagnóstico (*m.*)
diaper pañal (*m.*)
diaphragm diafragma (*m.*)
diarrhea diarrea (*f.*)
die morir (o:ue)
diet dieta (*f.*)
  go on a — seguir (e:i) una dieta
dietician dietista (*m., f.*)
different diferente, distinto(a)
difficult difícil
difficulty dificultad (*f.*)
digest digerir (e:ie)

digestive system aparato digestivo (*m.*)
dilated dilatado(a)
diminish disminuir; (*a pain*) aliviarse
dining room comedor (*m.*)
dinner cena (*f.*)
diphtheria difteria (*f.*)
diploma diploma (*m.*), título (*m.*)
direct dirigir
directly directamente
disability incapacidad (*f.*), defecto físico (*m.*)
disabled inválido(a)
discharge flujo (*m.*); (*from the hospital*) dar de alta
discipline disciplinar; disciplina (*f.*)
discomfort molestia (*f.*), malestar (*m.*)
discount descuento (*m.*)
discover descubrir
discrimination discriminación (*f.*)
discuss discutir
disease enfermedad (*f.*)
disfigure afear
disinfect desinfectar
disorder trastorno (*m.*)
disposable desechable
distinguish distinguir
diuretic diurético (*m.*)
dividend dividendo (*m.*)
divorce divorciarse
— **proceedings** trámites de divorcio (*m. pl.*)
divorced divorciado(a)
dizziness mareo (*m.*)
do hacer, realizar
doctor doctor(a) (*m., f.*), médico(a) (*m., f.*)
—**'s office** consultorio (*m.*)

document documento (*m.*)
dollar dólar (*m.*)
domestic violence violencia doméstica (*f.*)
donate donar
donor donante (*m., f.*)
door puerta (*f.*)
dosage dosis (*f.*)
dot punto (*m.*)
doubt duda (*f.*); dudar
down payment enganche (*m.*) (*Méx.*), entrada (*f.*), pago inicial (*m.*)
downtown area centro (*m.*)
drainage drenaje (*m.*)
dress vestido (*m.*)
drink beber, tomar; bebida (*f.*)
drive manejar, conducir, guiar (*Puerto Rico*)
drop gota (*f.*)
dropsy hidropesía (*f.*)
drug(s) droga(s) (*f.*)
 — addict drogadicto(a) (*m., f.*)
 become addicted to — endrogarse
 take — endrogarse, dar un viaje (*coll.*), tripear (*coll.*)
drunk driving manejar estando borracho(a) (en estado de embriaguez)
dry seco(a)
DT's delírium tremens (*m.*)
due to por
 — illness por enfermedad
dull (*pain*) sordo(a)
during durante
dye tinte (*m.*)

E

each cada
ear (*inner*) oído (*m.*), (*external*) oreja (*f.*)
  — canal conducto auditivo (*m.*), canal auditivo (*m.*)
  — drum tímpano (*m.*)
early temprano
earn ganar
earning ingreso (*m.*), ganancia (*f.*)
earthquake terremoto (*m.*)
easy fácil
eat comer
ecstasy éxtasis (*m.*)
eczema eccema (*m.*), eczema (*m.*)
effect efecto (*m.*)
effective efectivo(a), eficaz
egg huevo (*m.*), blanquillo (*m.*) (*Méx.*)
either tampoco
ejaculate eyacular
elastic elástico(a)
elbow codo (*m.*)
elderly man (woman) anciano(a) (*m., f.*), viejo(a) (*m., f.*)
electric(al) eléctrico(a)
  — appliance aparato eléctrico (*m.*), (equipo) electrodoméstico (*m.*)
  — outlet tomacorrientes (*m. sing.*), enchufe (*m.*)
  — plug cover enchufe de seguridad (*m.*)
electricity electricidad (*f.*)
electrocardiogram (EKG) electrocardiograma (*m.*)

electroencephalogram (EEG) electroencefalograma (*m.*)
elevated elevado(a)
elevator ascensor (*m.*), elevador (*m.*)
eligibility elegibilidad (*f.*)
eligible elegible
eliminate eliminar
else más
embolism embolia (*f.*)
emergency emergencia (*f.*)
  — room sala de emergencia (*f.*), sala de urgencia (*f.*)
emphysema enfisema (*f.*)
employ emplear
employee empleado(a) (*m., f.*)
empty vacío(a)
  with an — stomach en ayunas
enamel esmalte (*m.*)
endocrinologist endocrinólogo(a) (*m., f.*)
endometriosis endometrosis, endometriosis (*f.*)
endoscopy endoscopia, endoscopía (*f.*)
enema enema (*m.*), lavado intestinal (*m.*), lavativa (*f.*)
English (language) inglés (*m.*)
enough (lo) suficiente
enter entrar (en)
entrance entrada (*f.*)
entry entrada (*f.*)
epidemic epidemia (*f.*)
epilepsy epilepsia (*f.*)
equipment equipo (*m.*)
especially especialmente, sobre todo
estimate estimado (*m.*)
even aun

ever alguna vez
  hardly — casi nunca
every cada
  — . . . hours cada... horas
  — day todos los días
everything todo (*m.*)
  — possible todo lo posible
eviction desalojo (*m.*)
evil eye mal de ojo (*m.*)
ex ex
examination chequeo (*m.*), examen (*m.*)
examine chequear, examinar, reconocer
example ejemplo (*m.*)
excrement excremento (*m.*)
excuse me perdón
exempt exento(a)
exercise ejercicio (*m.*); hacer ejercicio
exhaustion cansancio (*m.*)
expense gasto (*m.*)
expensive caro(a)
expire vencer
explain explicar
expose (oneself) exponer(se)
expression expresión (*f.*)
extend extender (e:ie)
  — credit conceder un crédito
extra extra
extract sacar, extraer
extraction extracción (*f.*)
eye ojo (*m.*)
  — examination examen de la vista (*m.*)
eyebrow ceja (*f.*)
eyedropper gotero (*m.*), cuentagotas (*m. sing., pl.*)

eyeglasses anteojos (*m. pl.*), gafas (*f. pl.*), lentes (*m. pl.*), espejuelos (*m. pl.*) (*Cuba*)
eyelashes pestañas (*f.*)
eyelid párpado (*m.*)

F

face cara (*f.*)
— **down** boca abajo
— **up** boca arriba
factory fábrica (*f.*)
faint desmayarse, perder (e:ie) el conocimiento
fair justo(a)
faithfully fielmente
fall caer(se); otoño (*m.*)
— **down** caerse
— **ill** enfermarse
false postizo(a)
family familia (*f.*); (*adj.*) familiar
— **counselor** consejero(a) (*m., f.*)
— **room** sala de estar (*f.*)
— **tension** tensión familiar (*f.*)
far (away) lejos (de)
farewell despedida (*f.*)
farm worker trabajador(a) agrícola (*m., f.*)
farsighted présbite
farsightedness hiperopía (*f.*)
fast (*adj.*) rápido(a); (*adv.*) rápidamente
fasting en ayunas
fat grasa (*f.*); gordo(a)
father padre (*m.*), papá (*m.*)
— **-in-law** suegro (*m.*)
fatigue fatiga (*f.*)
fatty tissue tejido graso (*m.*)

favor favor (*m.*)
fear temer
feces materia fecal (*f.*)
federal federal
feed alimentar, dar de comer, amamantar
feel sentir(se) (e:ie)
— **better** aliviarse
— **sorry** arrepentirse (e:ie)
feet pies (*m. pl.*)
felony delito (*m.*)
female mujercita (*f.*) (*coll., Méx.*)
femur fémur (*m.*)
fertile fértil
fetus feto (*m.*)
fever fiebre (f.), calentura (*f.*)
few pocos(as)
fiber fibra (*f.*)
fibula fíbula (*f.*), peroné (*m.*)
field campo (*m.*)
file a law suit presentar una demanda
fill llenar
— **a tooth** emplomar, empastar
— **out (*forms*)** llenar
finally finalmente
finances finanzas (*f. pl.*)
financial económico(a)
— **assistance** ayuda en dinero (*f.*)
find encontrar (o:ue)
— **out** averiguar, enterarse
fine bueno, bien
—**, thank you. And you?** Bien, gracias. ¿Y Ud.?
finger dedo (*m.*)
finish terminar

fire incendio (*m.*); (*from a job*) despedir (e:i), cesantear
— **Department** Departamento de bomberos (*m.*)
first (*adj.*) primero(a); (*adv.*) antes, primero
— **aid** primeros auxilios (*m. pl.*)
— **aid kit** estuche de primeros auxilios (*m.*), botiquín de primeros auxilios (*m.*)
— **name** nombre de pila (*m.*)
the — thing lo primero
fish pescado (*m.*)
fist puño (*m.*)
fix arreglar
fixed fijo(a)
flatus flato (*m.*)
floor piso (*m.*)
floss (dental) hilo dental (*m.*), seda dental (*f.*)
flour harina (*f.*)
flu influenza (*f.*), gripe (*f.*)
fluoride fluoruro (*m.*)
fluoroscopy fluoroscopia, fluoroscopía (*f.*)
foam espuma (*f.*)
follow seguir (e:i)
following siguiente
the — lo siguiente
the — day al día siguiente
food alimento (*m.*), alimentación (*f.*), comida (*f.*)
— **stamp** estampilla para alimento (*f.*), cupón para comida (*m.*)
foot pie (*m.*)
for para, por
— **a few seconds** por unos segundos
— **a while** por un tiempo
— **example** por ejemplo

— **me (on my behalf)** por mí
— **that reason** por eso
— **today** para hoy mismo
— **what . . . ?** ¿para qué... ?
— **what reason?** ¿para qué?
forbid prohibir
force forzar (o:ue)
forceps fórceps (*m. sing., pl.*)
forehead frente (*f.*)
foreign extranjero(a)
foreigner extranjero(a) (*m., f.*)
forget olvidarse (de)
forgive perdonar
form planilla (*f.*), forma (*f.*) (*Méx.*)
formula fórmula (*f.*)
forward hacia adelante
foster: — **child** hijo(a) de crianza (*m., f.*)
— **home** hogar de crianza (*m.*), hogar sustituto (*m.*)
— **parents** padres de crianza (*m. pl.*)
fracture fractura (*f.*); fracturar(se), quebrarse (e:ie) (*Méx.*), romperse
free (of charge) (*adv.*) gratis; (*adj.*) gratuito(a)
— **service** servicio gratuito (*m.*)
— **time** rato libre (m.), tiempo libre (*m.*)
French fries papas fritas (*f. pl.*)
frequent frecuente
frequently con frecuencia
friend amigo(a) (*m., f.*)
fright susto (*m.*)
from de
fruit fruta (*f.*)
frustrated frustrado(a)
fuel combustible (*m.*)

full time (*adv.*) tiempo completo
funeral expenses gastos funerarios (*m. pl.*)
fungus hongo (*m.*)
furniture muebles (*m. pl.*)
  piece of — mueble (*m.*)
further más

G

gain ganancia (*f.*); ganar
  — weight subir de peso, aumentar de peso
gallbladder vesícula biliar (*f.*)
gallstones cálculos en la vesícula (*m. pl.*)
garage garaje (*m.*)
garden jardín (*m.*)
gardener jardinero(a) (*m., f.*)
gargle hacer gárgaras
gas gas (*m.*)
gasoline gasolina (*f.*)
gastritis gastritis (*f.*)
gauze gasa (*f.*)
general general
  — practitioner clínico (*m.*), internista (*m., f.*)
generally generalmente
genitals genitales (*m. pl.*)
gentleman señor (*m.*)
geriatrist geriatra (*m., f.*)
get conseguir (e:i), obtener
  — along well llevarse bien
  — better mejorarse
  — close acercarse
  — drunk emborracharse
  — even with desquitar(se)
  — hurt lastimarse

— **in touch** ponerse en contacto
— **married** casarse (con)
— **paid** cobrar
— **sick** enfermarse
¡— **well soon!** ¡Que se mejore!
gift regalo (*m.*)
girl niña (*f.*), muchacha (*f.*), mujercita (*f.*) (*coll., Méx.*)
girlfriend novia (*f.*)
give dar
— **a checkup** hacer un examen
— **a fine (ticket)** imponer una multa
— **a shot** poner una inyección
— **birth** dar a luz, parir
gland glándula (*f.*)
glans glande (*m.*)
glass vaso (*m.*)
little — vasito (*m.*)
glasses anteojos (*m. pl.*), lentes (*m. pl.*), gafas (*f. pl.*), espejuelos (*m. pl.*) (*Cuba*)
glaucoma glaucoma (*m.*)
gloves guantes (*m. pl.*)
go ir
— **around** andar
— **away** irse
— **down** bajar
— **in** entrar (en)
— **out (leave)** salir
— **through** atravesar
— **to bed** acostarse (o:ue)
— **up** subir
God grant ojalá, Dios quiera
goiter bocio (*m.*)
gonorrhea gonorrea (*f.*)

good bueno(a)
  — **afternoon.** Buenas tardes.
  — **evening (night).** Buenas noches.
  — **luck.** Buena suerte.
  — **morning (day).** Buenos días.
  — **night.** Buenas noches.
  It's a — thing! ¡Qué suerte!
good-bye adiós
grade grado (*m.*)
granddaughter nieta (*f.*)
grandfather abuelo (*m.*)
grandmother abuela (*f.*)
grandson nieto (*m.*)
grapefruit toronja (*f.*)
green verde
greenish verdoso(a)
greeting saludo (*m.*)
groin ingle (*f.*)
gross earnings entrada bruta (*f.*)
group grupo (*m.*)
guardian tutor(a) (*m., f.*)
gum (of mouth) encía (*f.*)
gunshot wound herida de bala (*f.*)
gurney camilla (*f.*)
gut tripa (*f.*), intestino (*m.*)
gynecologist ginecólogo(a) (*m., f.*)
gynecology ginecología (*f.*)

H

hair pelo (*m.*), cabello (*m.*)
half mitad (*f.*); (*adj.*) medio(a)
  — **an hour** media hora (*f.*)

— **brother (sister)** medio(a) hermano(a) (*m.*, *f.*)
hallucination alucinación (*f.*)
hallway pasillo (*m.*)
hamburger hamburguesa (*f.*)
hand mano (*f.*)
handbag bolsa (*f.*), cartera (*f.*)
handicapped incapacitado(a)
handwriting letra (*f.*)
happen pasar, ocurrir, suceder
hard duro(a)
hardening endurecimiento (*m.*)
hashish hachich (*m.*), hachís (*m.*)
hat gorro (*m.*)
have tener
— **a backache** tener dolor de espalda
— **a seat** tomar asiento
— **just (done something)** acabar de (+ *inf.*)
— **lunch** almorzar (o:ue)
— **surgery** operarse
— **the right to** tener derecho a
— **to (do something)** tener que (+ *inf.*)
— **worked** haber trabajado
hay fever fiebre de heno (*f.*)
head cabeza (*f.*)
— **of household** jefe(a) de familia (*m.*, *f.*), cabeza de la familia (*m.*, *f.*)
headache dolor de cabeza (*m.*)
health salud (*f.*)
— **Department** Departamento de Sanidad (*m.*)
— **insurance** seguro de salud (*m.*), aseguranza de salud (*f.*) (*Méx.*)
healthy sano(a), saludable

hear oír
hearing (court) audiencia (*f.*), vista (*f.*)
— **aid** audífono (*m.*)
— **test** examen del oído (*m.*)
heart corazón (*m.*)
— **attack** ataque al corazón (*m.*)
— **beat** latido (*m.*)
— **murmur** soplo cardíaco (*m.*)
— **transplant** trasplante de corazón (*m.*)
to have — trouble estar enfermo(a) del corazón, sufrir del corazón, padecer del corazón
heartburn acidez (*f.*)
heat calefacción (*f.*)
heat (up) calentar (e:ie)
heater calentador (*m.*), calentón (*m.*) (*Méx.*), estufa (*f.*)
heavy pesado(a)
heel talón (*m.*)
hello hola
help ayuda (*f.*); ayudar
helper asistente (*m., f.*)
hemorrhage hemorragia (*f.*)
hemorrhoids hemorroides (*f. pl.*), almorranas (*f. pl.*)
hepatitis hepatitis (*f.*)
her su(s)
here aquí
— **is** aquí tiene
— **it is.** Aquí está.
hereditary hereditario(a)
heroin heroína (*f.*), manteca (*f.*) (*coll., Caribe*)
herpes herpes (*m. sing.*)
high alto(a)

— **blood pressure** hipertensión (*f.*), presión alta (*f.*)
— **chair** sillita alta (*f.*)
hip cadera (*f.*)
his su(s)
hit pegar, golpear(se), dar golpes
HIV VIH (virus de inmunodeficiencia humana) (*m.*)
hives urticaria (*f.*), ronchas (*f. pl.*)
hoarse ronco(a)
hoarseness ronquera (*f.*)
hold aguantar
— **one's breath** aguantar la respiración
hole agujero (*m.*), hueco (*m.*)
holiday día feriado (*m.*), día de fiesta (*m.*)
home casa (*f.*), vivienda (*f.*)
— **for the elderly** asilo de ancianos (*m.*), casa para ancianos (*f.*)
homeless desalojado(a), sin hogar
honey miel (*f.*)
hope esperar
I — ojalá, Dios quiera
hose medias (*f. pl.*)
hospital hospital (*m.*), clínica (*f.*), policlínica (*f.*)
— **insurance** seguro de hospitalización (*m.*)
hospitalization hospitalización (*f.*)
hospitalized hospitalizado(a)
hot caliente
hour hora (*f.*)
hours horario (*m.*)
house casa (*f.*)
household: — **appliance** aparato eléctrico (*m.*), (equipo) electrodoméstico (*m.*)
— **expenses** gastos de la casa (*m. pl.*)

housekeeping quehaceres del hogar (de la casa) (*m. pl.*)
housewife ama de casa (*f.* but **el ama**)
housework trabajo de la casa (*m.*), tareas de la casa (*f. pl.*), quehaceres del hogar (de la casa) (*m. pl.*)
how como
how! ¡cómo!, ¡qué!
— **fortunate!** ¡Qué suerte!
how? ¿cómo?
— **about . . . ?** ¿Qué tal...?
— **are you?** ¿Cómo está Ud.?
— **are you feeling?** ¿Cómo se siente?
— **do you spell . . . ?** ¿Cómo se escribe ...?
— **frequently?** ¿Con qué frecuencia?
— **is it going?** ¿Qué tal?
— **long?** ¿cuánto tiempo?
— **long ago . . . ?** ¿Cuánto tiempo hace ...?
— **long have . . . ?** ¿Cuánto tiempo hace que... ?
— **long had . . . ?** ¿Cuánto tiempo hacía que... ?
— **many?** ¿cuántos(as)?
— **may I help you?** ¿En qué puedo servirle?
— **much?** ¿cuánto(a)?
— **much do you pay in rent?** ¿Cuánto paga de alquiler?
— **old are you?** ¿Cuántos años tiene Ud.?, ¿Qué edad tiene?
however sin embargo
human humano(a)
— **immunodeficiency virus (HIV)** virus de inmunodeficiencia humana (VIH) (*m.*)
humerus húmero (*m.*)

hungry: to be — tener hambre
hurt doler (o:ue), hacer daño
  — oneself lastimarse
husband esposo (*m.*), marido (*m.*)
hydrogen peroxide agua oxigenada (*f.* but **el agua**)
hygienist higienista (*m., f.*)
hypertension hipertensión (*f.*), presión alta (*f.*)
hypodermic syringe jeringuilla (*f.*), jeringa **hipodérmica** (*f.*)
hysterectomy histerectomía (*f.*)

I

I.V. serum suero (*m.*)
ice hielo (*m.*)
  — pack bolsa de hielo (*f.*)
idea idea (*f.*)
identification identificación (*f.*)
if si
  — only ojalá
  — possible si es posible
ilium hueso ilíaco (*m.*)
ill enfermo(a)
illegal immigrant inmigrante ilegal (*m., f.*), inmigrante indocumentado(a) (*m., f.*)
immediately inmediatamente
immigrant inmigrante (*m., f.*)
immigration inmigración (*f.*)
  — card tarjeta de inmigración (*f.*)
immunize vacunar
implant implante (*m.*)
importance importancia (*f.*)
important importante

impossible imposible
impotence impotencia (*f.*)
impotent impotente
improve mejorar
in en, dentro de
— **a hurry** de prisa
— **addition** además
— **addition to** además de
— **case of** en caso de
— **order to** para
— **that case** en ese caso
— **the morning (afternoon, evening)** por la mañana (tarde, noche), de la mañana (tarde, noche)
— **these situations** en estas situaciones
— **use** en uso
incapacitated incapacitado(a)
incest incesto (*m.*)
inch pulgada (*f.*)
incisor incisivo (*m.*)
include incluir
including incluido(a)
income entrada (*f.*), ingreso (*m.*)
— **tax** impuesto sobre la renta (*m.*)
increase aumento (*m.*); aumentar
increments of . . . dollars partidas de... dólares (*f. pl.*)
incubation incubación (*f.*)
incubator incubador (*m.*)
independent independiente
indicate indicar, señalar
inexpensive barato(a)
infect infectar
infection infección (*f.*)

infectious infeccioso(a)
inflammation inflamación (*f.*)
inflammatory inflamatorio(a)
influenza gripe (*f.*), monga (*f.*) (*coll., Puerto Rico*)
inform informar
information información (*f.*), datos (*m. pl.*)
inheritance herencia (*f.*)
initial inicial (*f.*)
initiate iniciar
inject (oneself) inyectar(se)
injection inyección (*f.*)
injured person herido(a) (*m., f.*)
injury herida (*f.*), lesión (*f.*)
ink tinta (*f.*)
inpatient paciente interno(a) (*m., f.*)
insanity locura (*f.*)
insecticide insecticida (*m.*)
insemination inseminación (*f.*)
insert insertar
inside adentro
  on the — por dentro
insomnia insomnio (*m.*)
instruction instrucción (*f.*)
instrument aparato (*m.*)
insulin insulina (*f.*)
insurance seguro (*m.*), aseguranza (*f.*) (*Méx.*)
  — company compañía de seguro (*f.*)
intensive intensivo(a)
  — care unit unidad de cuidados intensivos (*f.*)
interest interés (*m.*)
internal interno(a)
internist internista (*m., f.*), clínico (*m.*)

interview entrevista (*f.*); entrevistar
intestine intestino (*m.*)
  large — intestino grueso (*m.*)
  small — intestino delgado (*m.*)
intoxication intoxicación (*f.*)
intrauterine device (I.U.D.) aparato intrauterino (*m.*)
investigate investigar
investigator investigador(a) (*m., f.*)
investment inversión (*f.*)
iodine yodo (*m.*)
ipecac ipecacuana (*f.*)
iron hierro (*m.*), plancha (*f.*)
irritated irritado(a)
irritation irritación (*f.*)
It doesn't matter. No importa.
It is not that way. No es así.
it's (+ *time*) son las (+ *time*)
It's nobody's business. A nadie le importa.
itching comezón (*f.*), picazón (*f.*)
itself propio(a)

J

jacket chaqueta (*f.*), chamarra (*f.*) (*Méx.*)
jail cárcel (*f.*)
jaw (bone) mandíbula (*f.*), quijada (*f.*)
jelly jalea (*f.*)
jewelry joyas (*f. pl.*)
Jewish judío(a), hebreo(a)
job trabajo (*m.*), empleo (*m.*)
jobless desocupado(a)
joint (*drugs*) leño (*m.*), cucaracha (*f.*), porro (*m.*); (*anatomy*) articulación (*f.*)

judge juez(a) (*m., f.*)
juice jugo (*m.*)
just nada más que, no más que
to have — (done something) acabar de (+ *inf.*)
juvenile juvenil
— delinquent delincuente juvenil (*m., f.*)
— hall reclusorio para menores (*m.*)

K

keep mantener, quedarse con, guardar
— at hand tener a mano
— in mind tener en cuenta
kick patada (*f.*)
kidney riñón (*m.*)
— stones cálculos en el riñón (*m. pl.*), piedras en el riñón (*f. pl.*)
kill matar
killer joint porro mortal (*m.*)
kind amable
kitchen cocina (*f.*)
knee rodilla (*f.*)
knock at the door tocar a la puerta
know saber, conocer
I — it. Ya lo sé.
knowledge conocimiento (*m.*)
knuckle nudillo (*m.*)

L

labor parto (*m.*)
— pain dolor de parto (*m.*)
to be in — estar de parto

laboratory laboratorio (*m.*)
laborer obrero(a) (*m., f.*)
lady señora (*f.*)
lame cojo(a)
lamp lámpara (*f.*)
landlord (lady) dueño(a) de la casa (*m., f.*)
language idioma (*m.*)
laparoscopy laparoscopia, laparoscopía (*f.*)
large grande
laryngitis laringitis (*f.*)
last durar; (*adj.*) pasado(a), último(a)
  — name apellido (*m.*)
  — night anoche
  — time la última vez
late tarde
lately últimamente
later después, luego, más tarde
  — on más adelante
law ley (*f.*)
lawsuit demanda (*f.*)
lawyer abogado(a) (*m., f.*)
laxative purgante (*m.*), laxante (*m.*)
learn aprender
least: at — por lo menos
leave salir, irse, dejar
  — behind dejar
left izquierdo(a); izquierda (*f.*)
  to the — a la izquierda
leg pierna (*f.*)
lesion lesión (*f.*)
less menos
  — than menos que
  — than (+ *number*) menos de (+ *number*)
  — . . . than menos... que

let dejar
— (someone) know avisar, hacer saber
—'s see. A ver., Vamos a ver.
letter letra (*f.*); carta (*f.*)
leukemia leucemia (*f.*)
license licencia (*f.*)
driver's — licencia para conducir (*f.*)
lie mentira (*f.*); mentir (e:ie)
— down acostarse (o:ue)
life vida (*f.*)
— insurance seguro de vida (*m.*)
lift subir, levantar
light luz (*f.*); (*adj.*) ligero(a)
like como; gustar
— that así
— this así
limb extremidad (*f.*)
limitation limitación (*f.*)
limited limitado(a)
line (*on a paper or form*) línea (*f.*), renglón (*m.*); revestir (e:ie)
liniment linimento (*m.*)
lip labio (*m.*)
liquid líquido (*m.*)
list lista (*f.*)
little (*size*) pequeño(a); (*quantity*) poco(a); (*adv.*) poco
— by little poco a poco
a — un poco
live vivir
liver hígado (*m.*)
loan préstamo (*m.*)
local local
lodging vivienda (*f.*)

look mirar, verse
  — for buscar
long-term a largo plazo
lose perder (e:ie)
  — consciousness perder (e:ie) el conocimiento, desmayarse
  — weight adelgazar, bajar de peso, perder (e:ie) peso, rebajar
loss pérdida (*f.*)
lotion loción (*f.*)
loved one ser querido (*m.*)
low bajo(a)
  — fat con poca grasa
low-income (de) bajos ingresos
LSD ácido (*m.*)
lubricate lubricar
luck suerte (*f.*)
  What —! ¡Qué suerte!
luckily por suerte
lukewarm tibio(a)
lump bolita (*f.*), abultamiento (*m.*)
lunch almuerzo (*m.*), lonche (*m.*) (*coll., Méx.*), comida (*f.*)
lung pulmón (*m.*)
lymph gland ganglio linfático (*m.*)

M

M.D. doctor(a) (*m., f.*), médico(a) (*m., f.*)
ma'am señora (*f.*)
macaroni macarrones (*m. pl.*)
Madam señora (*f.*)
magazine revista (*f.*)
maiden name apellido de soltera (*m.*)

main principal
maintain mantener
major mayor
majority mayoría (*f.*)
make hacer
— **a decision** tomar una decisión
— **a false statement** hacer una declaración falsa
— **an appointment** pedir (e:i) turno, pedir (e:i) hora
— **better** mejorar
— **sure** asegurarse
— **violent** poner violento
makeup maquillaje (*m.*)
malaise malestar (*m.*)
malaria malaria (*f.*)
male varón (*m.*)
— **chauvinism** machismo (*m.*)
malignant maligno(a)
mammogram mamografía (*f.*)
man hombre (*m.*)
manifest manifestar (e:ie)
Many thanks. Muchas gracias.
many times muchas veces
margarine margarina (*f.*)
marijuana marihuana (*f.*), [*coll.:* yerba (*f.*), pito (*m.*), pasto (*m.*)]
marital status estado civil (*m.*)
mark marca (*f.*); marcar
market mercado (*m.*)
marriage matrimonio (*m.*)
— **certificate** certificado de matrimonio (*m.*), inscripción de matrimonio (*f.*), partida de matrimonio (*f.*)

married casado(a)
marry casarse (con)
mass masa (*f.*)
massage fricción (*f.*)
match fósforo (*m.*), cerillo (*f.*)
maternity ward sala de maternidad (*f.*)
matter importar
It doesn't —. No importa.
to not — no tener importancia
What's the — with you? ¿Qué te pasa?
mature madurar
may: it — be . . . puede ser
maybe a lo mejor, quizá(s)
meal comida (*f.*)
mean querer (e:ie) decir, significar
meantime: in the — mientras tanto
measles sarampión (*m.*)
measure medir (e:i)
meat carne (*f.*)
medical médico(a), clínico(a)
— history hoja clínica (*f.*), historia clínica (*f.*)
— insurance card tarjeta de seguro médico (*f.*)
medicated medicinal
medicinal medicinal
medicine medicina (*f.*), remedio (*m.*)
— chest (cabinet) botiquín (*m.*)
medium hard semiduro(a)
melon melón (*m.*)
member miembro (*m.*)
meningitis meningitis (*f.*)
menstruation menstruación (*f.*), regla (*f.*), periodo (*m.*)
mental mental

— **health** enfermedades mentales (*f. pl.*)
metatarsus metatarso (*m.*)
methadone metadona (*f.*)
method método (*m.*)
midday meal almuerzo (*m.*), comida (*f.*)
middle medio (*m.*)
— **name** segundo nombre (*m.*)
midwife partera (*f.*), comadrona (*f.*)
migraine migraña (*f.*)
milk leche (*f.*)
mine mío(a)
mineral mineral (*m.*)
minor menor, menor de edad
minute minuto (*m.*)
misbehave portarse mal
miscarriage malparto (*m.*), aborto espontáneo (*m.*), aborto natural (*m.*)
mischief travesura (*f.*)
mischievous travieso(a), majadero(a), juguetón(ona)
misdemeanor delito (*m.*)
Miss señorita (Srta.) (*f.*)
miss class faltar a clase
mistreat maltratar
mobile home casa rodante (*f.*)
model modelo (*m.*)
molar muela (*f.*), molar (*m.*)
mole lunar (*m.*)
mom madre (*f.*), mamá (*f.*)
moment momento (*m.*)
money dinero (*m.*)
monitored monitorizado(a)
month mes (*m.*)
monthly mensual, al mes

more más
  — or less más o menos
  — than (+ *number*) más de (+ *number*)
  — than ever más que nunca
  — . . . than más ... que
morning mañana (*f.*)
morphine morfina (*f.*)
mortgage hipoteca (*f.*)
mother madre (*f.*), mamá (*f.*)
  — -in-law suegra (*f.*)
mouse ratón (*m.*)
mouth boca (*f.*)
mouthwash enjuague (*m.*)
move mover(se) (o:ue); (*to another lodging*), mudarse; mudanza (*f.*)
Mr. señor (Sr.) (*m.*)
Mrs. señora (Sra.) (*f.*)
much (*adv.*) mucho
  too — demasiado
mucous membranes mucosas (*f. pl.*)
multiple sclerosis esclerosis múltiple (*f.*)
mumps paperas (*f. pl.*), farfallotas (*f. pl.*) (*coll., Puerto Rico*)
muscle músculo (*m.*)
must deber
  — (do something) deber (+ *inf.*)
mute mudo(a)
mutual fund fondo mutuo (*m.*)
my mi(s)
myself yo mismo(a)

N

name nombre (*m.*)

last — apellido (*m.*)
nape nuca (*f.*)
narrow estrecho(a)
nationality nacionalidad (*f.*)
natural healer curandero(a) (*m., f.*)
nanny niñera (*f.*)
nausea náusea (*f.*)
near cerca (de), cercano(a)
nearsighted miope, corto(a) de vista
nearsightedness miopía (*f.*)
necessarily necesariamente
necessary necesario(a)
neck cuello (*m.*), pescuezo (*m.*) (*coll.*)
need necesitar, hacer falta; necesidad (*f.*)
needle aguja (*f.*)
negative negativo(a)
neglect descuidar
neighbor vecino(a) (*m., f.*)
neighborhood barrio (*m.*)
neither tampoco
— . . . nor ni ... ni
nephew sobrino (*m.*)
nerve nervio (*m.*)
nervous nervioso(a)
— depression depresión nerviosa (*f.*)
net neto(a)
— income entrada neta (*f.*)
neurological neurológico(a)
neurologist neurólogo(a) (*m., f.*)
neurology neurología
never nunca
nevertheless sin embargo
new nuevo(a)
newborn baby recién nacido(a) (*m., f.*)

newlywed recién casado(a) (*m., f.*)
newspaper periódico (*m.*)
next próximo(a), siguiente
— **door** de al lado
— **one** el (la) próximo(a) (*m., f.*)
— **time** la próxima vez
— **week** la semana que viene, la semana próxima, la semana entrante
the — day al día siguiente
niece sobrina (*f.*)
night noche (*f.*)
— **before last** anteanoche
— **school** escuela nocturna (*f.*)
— **table** mesita de noche (*f.*)
nightgown camisón (*m.*)
nipple pezón (*m.*)
nitroglycerin nitroglicerina (*f.*)
no no, ningún(una)
— **longer** ya no
— **one** nadie
nobody nadie
noise ruido (*m.*)
none ninguno(a)
normal normal
normally normalmente
nose nariz (*f.*)
nostril ventana nasal (*f.*), ventana de la nariz (*f.*)
not no
— **a cent** ni un centavo
— **any** ningún(a)
— **at the present time** ahora no
— **go well** no andar bien
— **now** ahora no

note nota (*f.*)
nothing nada
notice notar
notify notificar
noun nombre (*m.*)
nourishment alimento (*m.*)
novocaine novocaína (*f.*)
now ahora, ahorita (*Méx.*), ya
numb entumecido(a); entumecer
number número (*m.*)
  phone — número de teléfono (*m.*)
numbered numerado(a)
numbness entumecimiento (m.)
nurse enfermero(a) (*m., f.*)
  — (a baby) dar el pecho, amamantar, dar de mamar
  —'s aide auxiliar de enfermera (*m., f.*)
nursery sala de bebés (*f.*)
  — school guardería (*f.*), centro de cuidado de niños (*m.*) (*Puerto Rico*)

O

obesity obesidad (*f.*), gordura (*f.*)
object objeto (*m.*)
obstetrician obstetra (*m., f.*)
obtain conseguir (e:i)
occupation ocupación (*f.*)
occur ocurrir
oculist oculista (*m., f.*)
odontologist odontólogo(a) (*m., f.*)
odor olor (*m.*)
  to have a bad — tener mal olor, apestar, tener peste

of de
  — age mayor de edad
  — course cómo no
offer brindar
office oficina (*f.*)
often a menudo
oh ah, ¡ay!
  — my goodness (God!)! ¡Ay, Dios mío!
oil aceite (*m.*)
oily grasiento(a)
ointment ungüento (*m.*)
okay bueno(a), Está bien.
old viejo(a)
older mayor
oldest el (la) mayor
on en, sobre
  — becoming (turning) . . . years old al cumplir ... años
  — (one's) side de lado
once una vez
oncologist oncólogo(a) (*m., f.*)
one uno(a)
  — hundred percent cien(to) por ciento
  the — who el (la) que
one-eyed tuerto(a)
one-handed manco(a)
one-legged cojo(a)
only (*adv.*) solamente, sólo; (*adj.*) único(a)
open abrir; abierto(a)
  — heart surgery operación de corazón abierto (*f.*)
opening entrada (*f.*)
operate operar

operating room sala de cirugía (*f.*), sala de operaciones (*f.*)
operation operación (*f.*)
ophthalmologist oculista (*m., f.*), oftalmólogo(a) (*m., f.*)
ophthalmology oftalmología (*f.*)
opium opio (*m.*)
opposite opuesto(a)
option opción (*f.*)
optometrist oculista (*m., f.*)
or o
oral bucal
orally por vía bucal, por vía oral
orange naranja (*f.*), anaranjado(a)
  — juice jugo de naranja (*m.*), jugo de china (*m.*) (*Puerto Rico*)
order orden (*f.*); ordenar
  in — to para
organ órgano (*m.*)
organization organización (*f.*)
original (*adj.*) original
originate provenir
orthodontia ortodoncia (*f.*)
orthodontist ortodoncista (*m., f.*)
orthopedic ortopédico(a)
orthopedist ortopedista (*m., f.*), ortopeda (*m., f.*)
other otro(a)
  the others los (las) demás (*m., f.*), los otros(as) (*m., f.*)
our nuestro(a)
out of order descompuesto(a)
  — reach fuera del alcance
  — the ordinary fuera de lo común
outpatient paciente externo(a) (*m., f.*)

outside afuera
on the — por fuera
ovary ovario (*m.*)
oven horno (*m.*)
over al dorso
overdose sobredosis (*f.*)
overweight exceso de peso (*m.*)
ovulation ovulación (*f.*)
ovum óvulo (*m.*)
owe deber
own propio(a); poseer
— a house tener casa propia
oxygen oxígeno (*m.*)

P

pacemaker marcapasos (*m. sing.*)
pacifier bobo (*m.*) (*Puerto Rico*), chupete (*m.*), chupón (*m.*) (*Méx.*), tete (*m.*) (*Cuba*)
pack bolsa (f.)
— of cigarettes cajetilla (*f.*)
page página (*f.*)
pain dolor (*m.*)
The — goes away. El dolor se me pasa.
painful doloroso(a)
painkiller pastilla para el dolor (*f.*), calmante (*m.*)
paint pintura (*f.*)
pair par (*m.*), pareja (*f.*)
pajamas pijama (*m.*)
pal compañero(a) (*m., f.*)
palate paladar (*m.*)
pale pálido(a)
palpitation palpitación (*f.*)

pamphlet folleto (*m.*)
pants pantalones (*m. pl.*)
pantyhose pantimedias (*f. pl.*)
Pap test (smear) examen Papanicolau (*m.*)
paper papel (*m.*)
papilloma papiloma (*m.*)
paralysis parálisis (*f.*)
paralyzed paralítico(a)
paramedic paramédico(a) (*m., f.*)
pardon perdonar
  — me perdón
parents padres (*m. pl.*)
  — helpline línea de ayuda a los padres (*f.*)
parking estacionamiento (*m.*)
parochial parroquial
part parte (*f.*)
partial parcial
participate participar
pass pasar, pasársele a uno
passbook libreta de ahorros (*f.*)
passport pasaporte (*m.*)
pasta pasta (*f.*)
pastor pastor(a) (*m., f.*)
patch mechón (*m.*)
patella rótula (*f.*)
patience paciencia (*f.*)
patient paciente (*m., f.*)
pay pagar
  — in installments pagar a plazos
payment pago (*m.*)
peach durazno (*m.*), melocotón (*m.*)
peanut butter mantequilla de maní (*f.*), mantequilla de cacahuete (*f.*)
pear pera (*f.*)

pediatrician pediatra (*m., f.*)
pediatrics pediatría (*f.*)
pelvic de la pelvis, pélvico(a)
penalty pena (*f.*), penalidad (*f.*)
pencil lápiz (*m.*)
penicillin penicilina (*f.*)
penis pene (*m.*), miembro (*m.*)
pension pensión (*f.*)
people gente (*f.*)
pepper chile (*m.*), pimiento (*m.*)
per day (week) por día (semana)
percent por ciento (*m.*)
perfect perfecto(a)
perfume perfume (*m.*)
perhaps a lo mejor, quizá(s), tal vez
period periodo (*m.*)
permanent permanente
permission permiso (*m.*)
perpetrate cometer
person persona (*f.*)
personal personal
personnel personal (*m.*)
pertussis tos ferina (*f.*)
phalange falange (*f.*)
pharmacy farmacia (*f.*), botica (*f.*), droguería (*f.*) (*in some L.A. countries*)
phlegm flema (*f.*)
phone teléfono (*m.*)
  — number número de teléfono (*m.*)
  to — llamar por teléfono
photocopy copia fotostática (*f.*), fotocopia (*f.*)
photograph fotografía (*f.*)
physical físico(a)
  — therapy terapia física (*f.*)

pie pastel (*m.*)
pill pastilla (*f.*), píldora (*f.*)
— **for pain** pastilla para el dolor (*f.*), calmante (*m.*)
pillow almohada (*f.*)
pimple grano (*m.*)
pineapple piña (*f.*)
pins and needles hormigueo (*m.*)
pint pinta (*f.*)
place colocar; lugar (*m.*)
— **of birth** lugar de nacimiento (*m.*)
— **of employment** lugar donde trabaja (*m.*)
placenta placenta (*f.*)
plan (to do something) pensar (e:ie) (+ *inf.*)
planning planificación (*f.*)
plaque placa (*f.*)
plastic plástico (*m.*)
play jugar (u:ue)
— **with fire** jugar con fuego
pleasant ameno(a)
please por favor, favor de (+ *inf.*)
pleasure gusto (*m.*)
pleuresy pleuresía (*f.*)
pneumonia pulmonía (*f.*), neumonía (*f.*)
podiatrist podiatra (*m., f.*)
poison veneno (*m.*); — (*oneself*) envenenar(se)
— **center** centro de envenenamiento (*m.*)
poisoning envenenamiento (*m.*)
police policía (*f.*)
police (force) policía (*f.*); (*officer*) policía (*m., f.*), agente de policía (*m., f.*)
policy póliza (*f.*)
polio(myelitis) polio, poliomielitis (*f.*)
pollen polen (*m.*)

poor pobre
— **little thing (one)** pobrecito(a) (*m., f.*)
porch portal (*m.*)
pore poro (*m.*)
portion porción (*f.*)
position posición (*f.*), cargo (*m.*)
positive positivo(a)
possibility posibilidad (*f.*)
possible posible
possibly posiblemente
post office oficina de correos (*f.*)
— **box** apartado postal (*m.*)
postal postal
— **code** zona postal (*f.*), código postal (*m.*) (*Méx.*)
postnatal postnatal
potato papa (*f.*)
pound libra (*f.*)
practice practicar
prank travesura (*f.*)
precaution precaución (*f.*)
prefer preferir (e:ie)
pregnancy embarazo (*m.*)
pregnant embarazada, encinta, preñada (*coll.*)
premature prematuro(a)
premium prima (*f.*)
prenatal prenatal
preparation preparación (*f.*)
prepare preparar
prescribe recetar
prescribed recetado(a)
prescription receta (*f.*)
present (*adj.*) actual; presentar; presente (*m.*), (*gift*) regalo (*m.*)

press apretar (e:ie)
pressure presión (*f.*)
pretty bonito(a)
prevent prevenir
previous anterior
prick pinchar
priest (Catholic) padre (*m.*), cura (*m.*), sacerdote (*m.*)
primary primario(a)
principal (at a school) director(a) de la escuela (*m., f.*)
print (printed letter) letra de imprenta (*f.*), letra de molde (*f.*)
printing letra de molde (*f.*)
prisoner preso(a) (*m., f.*)
private privado(a)
private parts partes privadas (*f. pl.*)
probable probable
probably probablemente
probation libertad condicional (*f.*)
problem problema (*m.*)
profession profesión (*f.*)
profit ganancia (*f.*)
program programa (*m.*)
prohibit prohibir
proof prueba (*f.*)
property propiedad (*f.*)
— **tax** impuesto sobre la propiedad (*m.*)
prostate gland próstata (*f.*)
prostatitis prostatitis (*f.*)
protect proteger
protein proteína (*f.*)
Protestant protestante
provide proporcionar

provisional provisional
psychiatric psiquiátrico(a)
psychiatry siquiatría (*f.*)
psychologist psicólogo(a) (*m., f.*)
psychosis sicosis (*f.*)
public público(a)
  notary — notario(a) público(a) (*m., f.*)
publish publicar
pull (teeth) sacar, extraer
pulp pulpa (*f.*)
pulse pulso (*m.*)
pump (the stomach) hacer un lavado de estómago
punch trompada (*f.*), puñetazo (*m.*)
punish castigar
pupil pupila (*f.*)
purgative purgante (*m.*)
purse bolsa (*f.*), cartera (*f.*)
pus supuración (*f.*), pus (*m.*)
push (*during labor*) pujar
put poner
  — a cast on enyesar, escayolar (*España*)
  — away guardar
  — in one's mouth meterse en la boca
  — on ponerse
  — to bed acostar (o:ue)
pyorrhea piorrea (*f.*)

Q

quack curandero
qualify calificar
quantity cantidad (*f.*)
quarter (*three months*) trimestre (*m.*); cuarto (*m.*)

— **of an hour** cuarto de hora (*m.*)
question pregunta (*f.*)
questionnaire cuestionario (*m.*)

R

rabbi rabí (*m.*), rabino (*m.*)
race raza (*f.*)
radiologist radiólogo(a) (*m., f.*)
radiology radiología (*f.*)
radius radio (*m.*)
railroad insurance seguro ferroviario (*m.*)
raincoat impermeable (*m.*), capa de agua (*f.*)
raise levantar
raising (upbringing) crianza (*f.*)
rapidly rápidamente
rare raro(a)
rash sarpullido (*m.*), erupción de la piel (*f.*)
react prender, reaccionar
read leer
ready listo(a)
real verdadero(a)
— **estate** bienes raíces (*m. pl.*), bienes inmuebles (*m. pl.*)
Really? ¿De veras?
receipt recibo (*m.*), comprobante (*m.*)
receive recibir
receptionist recepcionista (*m., f.*)
recertification recertificación (*f.*)
recipient recipiente (*m., f.*)
recognize reconocer
recommend recomendar (e:ie)
reconciliation reconciliación (*f.*)
records: medical — archivo clínico (*m.*)

recover recuperarse
recovery room sala de recuperación (*f.*)
rectum recto (*m.*)
red rojo(a)
— **Cross** Cruz Roja (*f.*)
reevaluate reevaluar
referral orden (*f.*)
reformatory reformatorio (*m.*)
refrigerator refrigerador (*m.*)
refund reembolso (*m.*)
refuse negarse (e:ie)
register matricularse
registration registro (*m.*), registración (*f.*) (*Méx.*), matrícula (*f.*)
regret arrepentirse (e:ie)
— **that . . .** sentir (e:ie) que
regularly regularmente
related relacionado(a)
relationship (in a family) parentesco (*m.*)
relative pariente (*m., f.*)
close — pariente cercano(a) (*m., f.*)
relax (oneself) relajarse
release (from hospital) dar de alta
remain quedarse
remainder resto (*m.*)
remember recordar (o:ue)
remove quitar
rent alquiler (*m.*), renta (*f.*)
repair reparación (*f.*)
report informe (*m.*), (*of a crime*) denuncia (*f.*); notificar, (*a crime*) denunciar
request pedir (e:i)
required requerido(a)
residence residencia (*f.*)

resident residente (*m., f.*)
resign renunciar
respiratory respiratorio(a)
responsible responsable
rest descansar; descanso (*m.*), (*remainder*) resto (*m.*)
restless travieso(a), majadero(a), juguetón(ona)
result resultado (*m.*)
  produce results dar resultado
retention retención (*f.*)
retina retina (*f.*)
retire jubilarse, retirarse
retired jubilado(a), pensionado(a), retirado(a)
retirement jubilación (*f.*), retiro (*m.*)
return regresar, volver (o:ue)
revenue ingreso (*m.*)
reverse reverso (*m.*)
review revisión (*f.*)
revival reanimación (*f.*)
rheumatic fever fiebre reumática (*f.*)
rheumatism reumatismo (*m.*)
rhythm ritmo (*m.*)
rib costilla (*f.*)
rice arroz (*m.*)
right (*law*) derecho (*m.*); (*direction*) derecha (*f.*); (*adj.*) derecho(a)
  —? ¿verdad?
  — away en seguida
  — here aquí mismo
  — now ahora mismo, ahorita (*Méx.*)
  That's —. Es cierto.
  to the — a la derecha
ring anillo (*m.*)
ringing (in the ear) ruido (*m.*)

rinse enjuagar
risk riesgo (*m.*); arriesgar
robe bata (*f.*)
roll up one's sleeve(s) subirse la(s) manga(s), remangarse
room cuarto (*m.*), espacio (*m.*), habitación (*f.*), sala (*f.*)
— **and board** el alojamiento y las comidas (*m.*)
— **temperature** temperatura del ambiente (*f.*)
root raíz (*f.*)
— **canal** canal en la raíz (*m.*)
roughage fibras (*f. pl.*)
routinely de rutina
rub fricción (*f.*); friccionar
rubella rubéola (*f.*)
rug alfombra (*f.*)
rule reglamento (*m.*)
rump nalga (*f.*)
run correr
in the long — a la larga
— **a test** hacer un análisis, hacer una prueba
— **into** chocar

S

safe caja de seguridad (*f.*), caja fuerte (*f.*); (*adj.*) seguro(a)
safety cap (cover) tapa de seguridad (*f.*)
salary sueldo (*m.*), salario (*m.*)
saliva saliva (*f.*)
salt sal (*f.*)
— **free** sin sal
same mismo(a)

the — lo mismo
the — as before el (la) mismo(a) de antes
sample muestra (*f.*)
save guardar, salvar
savings account cuenta de ahorros (*f.*)
say decir (e:i)
scab costra (*f.*)
scabies sarna (*f.*)
scalp cuero cabelludo (*m.*)
scapula omóplato (*m.*)
scar cicatriz (*f.*)
scarf bufanda (*f.*)
scarlet fever fiebre escarlatina (*f.*)
schedule horario (*m.*)
schizophrenia esquizofrenia (*f.*)
scholarship beca (*f.*)
school escuela (*f.*)
scissors tijeras (*f. pl.*)
security deposit depósito de seguridad (*m.*)
scratch rasguño (*m.*); rascar(se)
scrotum escroto (*m.*)
seat: Have a —. Tome asiento.
second segundo (*m.*); segundo(a)
secondary school (junior and high school) escuela secundaria (*f.*)
secretion secreción (*f.*)
section sección (*f.*)
sedative calmante (*m.*), sedante (*m.*), sedativo (*m.*)
see ver
— you tomorrow. Hasta mañana.
seem parecer, verse
seizure ataque (*m.*)
select elegir (e:i)

self-employed: to be — trabajar por su cuenta, trabajar por cuenta propia
sell vender
semen semen (*m.*)
semester semestre (*m.*)
seminal vesicle vesícula seminal (*f.*)
semiprivate semiprivado(a)
send mandar, enviar
senses sentidos (*m. pl.*)
separate separar
separated separado(a)
separation separación (*f.*)
serious grave, serio(a)
servant sirviente (*m., f.*)
serve servir (e:i)
service servicio (*m.*)
 — station estación de servicio (*f.*), gasolinera (*f.*)
several varios(as)
sex sexo (*m.*)
 to have — tener relaciones sexuales, acostarse con
sexual sexual
 — abuse abuso sexual (*m.*)
 — partner compañero(a) sexual (*m., f.*)
 — relations relaciones sexuales (*f. pl.*)
sexually a través del contacto sexual
shaded sombreado
shaking temblor (*m.*)
share compartir; (*of stock*) acción (*f.*)
sharp agudo(a), punzante
 — pain punzada (*f.*)
shave afeitar(se), rasurar(se)
shirt camisa (*f.*)

shoe zapato (*m.*)
shoot dar un tiro, pegar un tiro
  — up pullar (*Caribe*)
shop tienda (*f.*)
short breve; (*length*) corto(a); (*height*) bajo(a)
  to be — of breath faltarle el aire a uno
shot inyección (*f.*)
should (do something) deber (+ *inf.*)
shoulder hombro (*m.*)
sick enfermo(a)
sick person enfermo(a) (*m., f.*)
sickness enfermedad (*f.*)
side lado (*m.*), costado (*m.*)
  at the — of al lado de
  — effect efecto secundario (*m.*)
  to (at) the sides a los costados, a los lados
sign firmar; señal (*f.*)
signature firma (*f.*)
similar similar
simple simple
simply simplemente
since como, desde
single soltero(a)
sir señor (*m.*)
sister hermana (*f.*)
  — -in-law cuñada (*f.*)
sit sentar(se) (e:ie)
  — down. Siéntese.
  — still quedarse quieto(a)
sitting sentado(a)
situation situación (*f.*)
sixth sexto(a)
size tamaño (*m.*)

skeleton esqueleto (*m.*)
skim milk leche descremada (*f.*)
skin piel (*f.*); (*face*) cutis (*m.*)
skirt falda (*f.*)
skull cráneo (*m.*)
slap bofetada (*f.*), galleta (*f.*) (*Cuba y Puerto Rico*)
sleep dormir (o:ue)
sleeve manga (*f.*)
slip resbalar
slipper zapatilla (*f.*), babucha (*f.*)
slowly despacio, lentamente
small pequeño(a)
— **truck** camioncito (*m.*)
smallpox viruela (*f.*)
smoke fumar; humo (*m.*)
smoked ahumado(a)
so así que, así
— **long** tanto tiempo
— **many** tantos(as)
— **much** tanto(a)
— **that** de modo que
soap jabón (*m.*)
social social
— **Security** Seguro Social (*m.*)
— **Security card** tarjeta de Seguro Social (*f.*)
— **services** asistencia social (*f.*)
— **Welfare Department** Departamento de Bienestar Social (*m.*)
— **worker** trabajador(a) social (*m., f.*)
— **worker (who makes home visits)** visitador(a) social (*m., f.*)
socket tomacorrientes (*m. sing.*), enchufe (*m.*)

socks calcetines (*m. pl.*), medias de hombre (*f. pl.*), tobilleras (*f. pl.*) (*Méx.*)
soda pop refresco (*m.*)
sofa sofá (*m.*)
soft blando(a)
  — drink refresco (*m.*)
sole (of foot) planta del pie (*f.*)
solve resolver (o:ue)
some algún, alguna; algunos(as)
somebody alguien
someone alguien
  — else otra persona (*f.*)
something algo (*m.*)
sometimes algunas veces, a veces
son hijo (*m.*)
  — -in-law yerno (*m.*)
sonogram sonograma (*m.*)
soon pronto
  as — as en cuanto, tan pronto como
sooner: the —, the better en cuanto antes mejor
sore llaga (*f.*)
  — throat dolor de garganta (*m.*)
sorry: I'm —. Lo siento.
soup sopa (*f.*)
source fuente (*f.*)
  — of income fuente de ingreso (*f.*)
space espacio (*m.*)
spaghetti espaguetis (*m. pl.*)
Spanish (language) español (*m.*)
spanking paliza (*f.*), nalgada (*f.*)
speak hablar
special especial
specialist especialista (*m., f.*)
specify especificar

specimen muestra (*f.*)
speech impediment dificultad del habla (*f.*)
spend (*money*) gastar; (*time*) pasar
sperm esperma (*f.*)
spiced condimentado(a)
spicy picante, condimentado(a)
spinal anesthesia raquídea (*f.*)
spine (spinal column) columna vertebral (*f.*), espina dorsal (*f.*)
spit escupir
spleen bazo (*m.*)
sponge esponja (*f.*)
  — bath baño de esponja (*m.*)
spoonful cucharada (*f.*)
spring primavera (*f.*)
sputum esputo (*m.*)
stab dar una puñalada
stabbing agudo(a), punzante
staff personal (*m.*)
staircase escalera (*f.*)
stairs escalera (*f.*)
stand pararse, aguantar
  — up pararse
start comenzar (e:ie), empezar (e:ie)
starting with a partir de
state estado (*m.*); (*adj.*) estatal
stay quedarse
step paso (*m.*)
stepbrother hermanastro (*m.*)
stepchild hijastro(a) (*m.*, *f.*)
stepfather padrastro (*m.*)
stepmother madrastra (*f.*)
stepsister hermanastra (*f.*)
sterility esterilidad (*f.*)

sterilize esterilizar
sternum esternón (*m.*)
stick out (one's tongue) sacar (la lengua)
still todavía
  to keep — quedarse quieto(a)
stitch punto (*m.*), puntada (*f.*)
stock acción (*f.*)
stockings medias (*f. pl.*)
  support — medias elásticas (*f. pl.*)
stomach estómago (*m.*), barriga (*f.*)
stomachache dolor de estómago (*m.*)
stone cálculo (*m.*), piedra (*f.*)
stool materia fecal (*f.*), caca (*f.*) (*coll.*)
  — specimen muestra de heces fecales (*f.*), muestra de excremento (*f.*)
stop detener
  — (doing something) dejar de (+ *inf.*)
storage almacenaje (*m.*)
stove cocina (*f.*), estufa (*f.*), fogón (*m.*)
straight directamente
strange (unknown) extraño(a)
stranger persona extraña (*f.*)
strawberry fresa (*f.*)
street calle (*f.*)
strenuous violento(a)
stress estrés (*m.*)
stretch extender (e:ie)
stretcher camilla (*f.*)
strict estricto(a)
strike pegar, golpear, dar golpes
stroke derrame (*m.*), embolia (*f.*), hemorragia cerebral (*f.*)
strong fuerte
student visa visa de estudiante (*f.*)

study estudiar
— a language tomar un idioma
sty orzuelo (*m.*)
subscription suscripción (*f.*)
subsidy subsidio (*m.*), subvención (*f.*)
sue demandar
suffer sufrir, padecer
sufficient suficiente
suffocate (oneself) asfixiar(se), sofocar(se)
sugar azúcar (*m.* or *f.*)
suggest sugerir (e:ie)
suggestion sugerencia (*f.*)
sulfa sulfa (*f.*)
summary resumen (*m.*)
summer verano (*m.*)
sun sol (*m.*)
sunstroke insolación (*f.*)
supervisor supervisor(a) (*m., f.*)
supper cena (*f.*)
supplemental suplementario(a)
support (oneself) mantener(se) (e:ie)
suppository supositorio (*m.*)
sure seguro(a)
—! ¡Cómo no!
make — asegurarse
surgeon cirujano(a) (*m., f.*)
surgery cirugía (*f.*), operación (*f.*)
surgical quirúrgico(a)
surname apellido (*m.*)
suspect sospechar
suspicion sospecha (*f.*)
swallow tragar
sweat sudar
sweet caramelo (*m.*), dulce (*m.*); (*adj.*) dulce

sweetened endulzado(a)
swelling inflamación (*f.*), hinchazón (*f.*)
swimming pool piscina (*f.*), alberca (*f.*) (*Méx.*)
swollen hinchado(a), inflamado(a)
symptom síntoma (*m.*)
synagogue sinagoga (*f.*)
syphilis sífilis (*f.*); (*adj.*) sifilítico(a)
syringe jeringa (*f.*), jeringuilla (*f.*)
syrup jarabe (*m.*)

T

table mesa (*f.*)
tablespoonful cucharada (*f.*)
tablet tableta (*f.*), pastilla (*f.*)
tachycardia taquicardia (*f.*)
take llevar, tomar, agarrar, coger
— **away** quitar
— **care of** atender (e:ie), cuidar; (of oneself) cuidarse
— **note** anotar
— **off one's clothes** quitar(se) la ropa
— **out** sacar, extraer, quitar
— **part** participar
— **(someone or something somewhere)** llevar
— **the blood pressure** tomar la presión, tomar la tensión
— **(time)** demorar
talk conversar, hablar
tall alto(a)
How — are you? ¿Cuánto mide Ud.?
tarsus tarso (*m.*)
tartar sarro (*m.*)

tax impuesto (*m.*)
taxpayer contribuyente (*m., f.*)
tea té (*m.*)
teacher maestro(a) (*m., f.*)
tear duct conducto lacrimal (*m.*), conducto lagrimal (*m.*)
teaspoonful cucharadita (*f.*)
technician técnico (*m., f.*)
teenager adolescente (*m., f.*)
teeth (set of teeth) dentadura (*f.*)
telephone teléfono (*m.*)
— **book** guía telefónica (*f.*), directorio telefónico (*m.*)
— **number** número de teléfono (*m.*)
television televisión (*f.*)
— **set** televisor (*m.*)
tell decir (e:i), informar
— **a lie** mentir (e:ie)
temperature temperatura (*f.*)
temple sien (*f.*), sinagoga (*f.*)
temporary temporal
tend atender (e:ie)
tendency tendencia (*f.*)
tense up ponerse tenso(a)
tension tensión (*f.*)
tepid tibio(a)
term plazo (*m.*), término (*m.*)
terrible terrible
test análisis (*m.*), prueba (*f.*)
test tube probeta (*f.*)
testicle testículo (*m.*)
tetanus tétano(s) (*m.*)
— **shot** inyección contra el tétano (*f.*), inyección antitetánica (*f.*)

textbook libro de texto (*m.*)
thank agradecer
— you (very much). (Muchas) Gracias.
— goodness! ¡Qué bueno!, menos mal
that que, eso
— is to say . . . Es decir...
— way así
— which lo que
—'s all. Eso es todo.
—'s fine. Está bien.
—'s great! ¡Qué bueno!
—'s why por eso
their su
then entonces, luego
therapy terapia (*f.*)
there allí
— is (are) hay
— is going to be va a haber
— are (+ *number*) of us. Somos (+ *number*).
— was había
thermometer termómetro (*m.*)
these estos(as)
— days en estos días
thigh muslo (*m.*)
thin delgado(a)
thing cosa (*f.*)
think creer, pensar (e:ie)
— about that pensar (e:ie) en eso
— so creer que sí
not — so creer que no
third tercero(a)
thirst sed (*f.*)
this este(a)
— one éste(a) (*m., f.*)

— **very day** hoy mismo
thorax tórax (*m.*)
those aquéllos(as) (*m., f.*)
throat garganta (*f.*)
through por
— **the mouth** por la boca
throw up vomitar, arrojar
thyroid tiroides (*m. sing.*)
tibia tibia (*f.*)
tie ligar, amarrar
— **the tubes** ligar los tubos, amarrar los tubos
tightness opresión (*f.*)
till hasta
time (*in a series*) vez (*f.*); tiempo (*m.*)
at the present — actualmente
from — **to** — de vez en cuando
many times muchas veces
on — a tiempo
tired cansado(a)
tiredness cansancio (*m.*)
tissue tejido (*m.*), pañuelo de papel (*m.*)
title título (*m.*)
to para, a
— **see if . . .** para ver si...
toast tostada (*f.*), pan tostado (*m.*)
tobacco tabaco (*m.*)
today hoy
—**'s date** fecha de hoy (*f.*)
toe dedo del pie (*m.*)
big — dedo gordo (*m.*)
together junto(a)
toilet inodoro (*m.*)
tolerate aguantar

tomato tomate (*m.*)
tomorrow mañana
the day after — pasado mañana (*m.*)
tongue lengua (*f.*)
tonsilitis amigdalitis (*f.*)
tonsils amígdalas (*f. pl.*)
too much demasiado(a)
tooth diente (*m.*), muela (*f.*)
toothbrush cepillo de dientes (*m.*)
toothpaste pasta dentífrica (*f.*), pasta de dientes (*f.*)
tortilla tortilla (*f.*)
total total
touch tocar
tourniquet ligadura (*f.*), torniquete (*m.*)
trade oficio (*m.*)
training entrenamiento (*m.*), capacitación (*f.*)
tranquilizer sedante (*m.*), tranquilizante (*m.*)
transfusion transfusión (*f.*)
transgression of law delito (*m.*)
translator traductor(a) (*m., f.*)
transmitted trasmitido(a)
transportation transportación (*f.*)
treat tratar
treatment tratamiento (*m.*)
tree árbol (*m.*)
tremor temblor (*m.*)
trimester trimestre (*m.*)
trouble molestia (*f.*)
trousers pantalones (*m. pl.*)
true verdad, verdadero(a)
try probar (o:ue), tratar (de)
T-shirt camiseta (*f.*)
tube tubo (*m.*)

tuberculin tuberculina (*f.*)
tuberculosis tuberculosis (*f.*)
tumor tumor (*m.*)
turn ponerse
 — **blue** ponerse azul
 — **pale** ponerse pálido(a)
 — **out okay** salir bien
 — **over** volverse (o:ue), darse vuelta, voltearse (*Méx.*)
 — **red** ponerse rojo(a)
 — **white** ponerse blanco(a)
 — **to** recurrir (a)
TV televisor (*m.*)
tweezers pinzas (*f. pl.*)
twins mellizos(as) (*m. pl., f. pl.*), gemelos(as) (*m. pl., f. pl.*), cuates (*m. pl., f. pl.*) (*Méx.*), jimaguas (*m. pl., f. pl.*) (*Cuba*)
twist torcer(se) (o:ue)
twitching temblor (*m.*)
type tipo (*m.*); escribir a máquina

U

ulcer úlcera (*f.*)
ulna cúbito (*m.*)
ultrasound ultrasonido (*m.*), ultrasonografía (*f.*)
umbilical cord cordón umbilical (*m.*)
unable to work incapacitado(a) para trabajar
unbearable insoportable
uncle tío (*m.*)
under debajo (de), bajo
underwear ropa interior (*f.*)
undress desvestir(se) (e:i)

unfortunately por desgracia, desgraciadamente
unit unidad (*f.*)
until hasta (que)
— **recently** hasta hace poco
upset disgustado(a)
uremia uremia (*f.*), urea alta (*f.*)
urethra uretra (*f.*), canal de la orina (*m.*), caño de la orina (*m.*)
urgent urgente
urgently urgentemente
uric úrico(a)
urinate orinar
urine orina (*f.*)
— **specimen** muestra de orina (*f.*)
urologist urólogo(a) (*m.*, *f.*)
urology urología (*f.*)
us nosotros(as) (*m.*, *f.*)
use utilizar, usar
used usado(a)
useful útil
uterus útero (*m.*)
uvula campanilla (*f.*), úvula (*f.*)

V

vacate desocupar, desalojar
vaccinate vacunar
vaccinated vacunado(a)
vaccine vacuna (*f.*)
vagina vagina (*f.*)
vaginal vaginal
vaginitis vaginitis (*f.*)
value valor (*m.*)

varicose veins várices (*f. pl.*), venas varicosas (*f. pl.*)
variety variedad (*f.*)
vasectomy vasectomía (*f.*)
Vaseline vaselina (*f.*)
vegetable vegetal (*m.*), legumbre (*f.*)
vein vena (*f.*)
venereal venéreo(a)
verb verbo (*m.*)
verification verificación (*f.*)
verify verificar
vertebra vértebra (*f.*)
very muy
  — kind (of you) muy amable
  — much muchísimo(a)
  (Not) — well. (No) Muy bien.
vesicle vesícula (*f.*)
victim víctima (*f.*)
view vista (*f.*)
violent violento(a)
virus virus (*m.*)
vision vista (*f.*)
visit visitar
visitation rights derecho a visitar (*m.*)
visiting hours horas de visita (*f. pl.*)
visiting nurse enfermero(a) visitador(a) (*m., f.*)
vitamin vitamina (*f.*)
vocabulary vocabulario (*m.*)
vocational vocacional
  — training reorientación vocacional (*f.*)
vomit arrojar, vomitar

W

waist cintura (*f.*)
wait esperar
  — on atender (e:ie)
waiting room sala de espera (*f.*)
waive renunciar
wake (someone up) despertar (e:ie)
  — up despertarse (e:ie)
walk caminar, andar
walker andador (*m.*)
wall pared (*f.*)
want desear, querer (e:ie)
ward sala (*f.*)
warn avisar, hacer saber
warning aviso (*m.*)
warrant orden de detención (*f.*), permiso de detención (*m.*)
wart verruga (*f.*)
washcloth toallita (*f.*)
washing lavado (*m.*)
watch reloj (*m.*)
water agua (*f.*)
  — bag bolsa de agua (*f.*)
way forma (*f.*), manera (*f.*)
  It is not that —. No es así.
  that — así
weak débil
weakness debilidad (*f.*)
wear usar
week semana (*f.*)
weekend fin de semana (*m.*)
weekly (*adj.*) semanal; (*adv.*) semanalmente, por semana

weigh pesar
weight peso (*m.*)
welcome: You're —. De nada., No hay de qué.
well bien, bueno, pues
what cuál, qué, lo que
what? ¿qué?, ¿cuál?
  — can I do for you? ¿En qué puedo servirle (ayudarle)?, ¿Qué se le ofrece?
  — do you (does he/she) need? ¿Qué necesita?
  — for? ¿Para qué?
  —'s happening? ¿Qué pasa?
  — time? ¿a qué hora?
  — time is it? ¿Qué hora es?
wheelchair silla de ruedas (*f.*)
when cuando
when? ¿cuándo?
where donde
where? ¿dónde?
  — (to)? ¿adónde?
  to — ? ¿adónde? (¿a dónde?)
which ¿cuál?
while mientras; rato (*m.*)
  a — later al rato
white blanco(a)
who quien
who? ¿quién?
whom? ¿quién?
whooping cough tos ferina (*f.*), tos convulsiva (*f.*)
why? ¿para qué?, ¿por qué?
widow viuda (*f.*)
widower viudo (*m.*)
wife esposa (*f.*), mujer (*f.*), señora (*f.*)

window ventana (*f.*)
windshield parabrisas (*m.*)
wine vino (*m.*)
winter invierno (*m.*)
wisdom tooth muela del juicio (*f.*), cordal (*m.*)
wish desear, querer (e:ie)
with con
— **her** con ella
— **me** conmigo
withdraw retirarse
within dentro de
— **reach** a su alcance
without sin
— **cost** gratis
— **fail** sin falta
witness testigo (*m.*, *f.*)
woman mujer (*f.*)
womb matriz (*f.*)
wonderful maravilloso(a)
word palabra (*f.*)
work trabajo (*m.*); trabajar, dar resultado
— **full-time** trabajar tiempo completo
— **part-time** trabajar parte del tiempo, trabajar medio día
— **permit** permiso de trabajo (*m.*)
worker obrero(a) (*m.*, *f.*), trabajador(a) (*m.*, *f.*)
—**'s compensation** compensación obrera (*f.*)
worried preocupado(a)
worry (about) preocupar(se) por
worse peor
worst peor
wound herida (*f.*), llaga (*f.*)
wounded herido(a)
wrist muñeca (*f.*)

write escribir
  — down anotar
written escrito(a)

X

X (letter of alphabet) equis (*f.*)
X-ray radiografía (*f.*)
  — room sala de rayos X (*f.*)

Y

year año (*m.*)
yearly (*adv.*) al año; (*adj.*) anual
yellow amarillo(a)
yellowish amarillento(a)
yes sí
yesterday ayer
yet todavía
yogurt yogur (*m.*)
young joven
  — lady señorita (*f.*)
  — man muchacho (*m.*)
  — woman muchacha (*f.*)
younger menor
youngest el (la) menor
your su(s)
You're welcome. De nada., No hay de qué.
yours suyo(a)

Z

zip code zona postal (*f.*), código postal (*m.*) (*Méx.*)